# BRENDA WATSON'S
# NATURAL PET CARE
## FOR **DOGS** LONG LIFE FOR YOUR BEST FRIEND

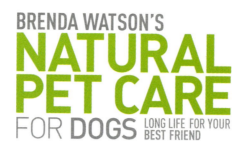

# BRENDA WATSON'S NATURAL PET CARE FOR DOGS
## LONG LIFE FOR YOUR BEST FRIEND

**By Brenda Watson**
**With Dr. Joel Murphy**
**and Jemma Sinclaire D.C.**

**ISBN 978-0-692-99734-5**

This book is for educational purposes. It is not intended as a substitute for medical advice. Please consult a qualified health care professional for individual health and medical advice. Neither Brenda Watson Media nor the author shall have any responsibility for any adverse effects arising directly or indirectly as a result of the information provided in this book. Throughout this book, trademarked names are used. Rather than put a trademark symbol after every occurrence of a trademarked name, we use names in an editorial fashion only, and to the benefit of the trademark owner, with no intention of infringement of the trademark. Where such designations appear in this book, they have been printed with initial caps.

**Book Design:** Paul Pavlovich
**Photos courtesy of Shutterstock.com**

**Brenda Watson Media**
133 Candy Lane
Palm Harbor, FL
34683

# ACKNOWLEDGEMENTS

The gratitude and thanks I feel for all the teachers in my life goes beyond anything I could list here. The 25 years I have spent in the human health industry has led me to the path of now helping our pets have a life of longevity and good health. These furry friends who bring unconditional love into our hearts is the most inspiring new focus in my life.

Thank you, Stan Watson, my husband, for leading me to this path of helping pets to enjoy a better life through diet and supplementation. Your love of animals has made the transition from human health to pet health so natural for both of us.

Many thanks to Dr. Joel Murphy for your experience and guidance over the last 20 years as you have led us in knowing that what we need as humans to help us age gracefully are the same things that support our dogs and cats in vitality as well. You are an amazing Veterinarian and I am blessed to have worked with you over these years.

A special thanks to Jemma Sinclaire. Without her this book would not have come to fruition. Your love of the animal world aligns with all Vital Planet stands for.

To my special family - Chris, Joy, Ella and Ava - I thank you for your loving support as we build a company dedicated to helping our world. Your support for me is instrumental in our mission at Vital Planet.

A special thanks to Brenda Valen for her continued support all these years as we embark on this new mission. You have always stood by me with your brilliant mind and practicality that is always needed and greatly appreciated.

A very big "Thank You" to everyone at Vital Planet for your passion and persistence in getting our message out to the world. Together we will make pet health through diet and supplementation every household's goal – so they will enjoy the maximum number of years with their happy and vital dog!

Sincerely

Brenda Watson

# BRENDA WATSON BIO

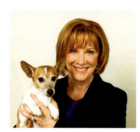

For more than 25 years, Brenda Watson, C.N.C, has helped people achieve vibrant, lasting health through improved digestive function. Her knowledge is surpassed only by her enthusiasm and ability to engage her audience – whatever the medium.

As a New York Times best-selling author with seven books completed to date, the Diva of Digestion continues to educate people about how digestive health is the foundation upon which total-body health is built. Brenda's high-energy, no-nonsense approach to bodily functions has made her a popular presenter on PBS and a frequent health expert on national television. In fact, she was recently seen as an expert on the newly popular Pet Talk on the National Geographic Wild channel

Recently, Brenda has turned her focus onto another very important matter, the health of your pets, and her own. Brenda believes that just like us humans, your dog and cat's digestive system can be the root cause of many health issues. And having a proper balance of intestinal bacteria and a healthy digestive system is an essential part of maintaining overall health in your pet.

Brenda is confident the information in this book will help you create a life of full of love and longevity in your companion animals. Knowledge is power.

# JEMMA SINCLAIRE BIO

A Chiropractic Physician and Nutritionist by trade, Jemma Sinclaire, has dedicated her adult life to the art of healing from the inside out. After, and ironically, a spinal injury limited her ability to practice Chiropractic she turned her attention to her second love, research and writing.

Meeting Brenda Watson in 2010 was a turning point in her life. Jemma began a career of assisting Brenda with researching and writing her last three books as well as her very popular Public Television shows revolving around human health and wellness. When Brenda Watson changed her focus to the health and wellness of our pets Jemma was fully on board. Jemma's love of animals has now found a productive outlet as she has always felt her true vocational calling in life was that of a veterinarian. Jemma's in-depth understanding of human neurology, anatomy and physiology has transferred over into her ability to understand and write on the health of our pets.

Jemma's sincere hope is that whoever reads this book learns something that will add years of joy to the wonderful relationship they have with their dog, their best friend

# A LITTLE ABOUT
# DR. JOEL MURPHY

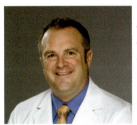

Dr. Murphy has never been satisfied with being average at what he does. He has created a whole new standard in veterinary care. The Animal & Bird Medical Center of Palm Harbor, Florida, a full-service hospital and boarding center, reflects his continued effort to offer his clients a higher standard in care for their cherished pets.

Dr. Murphy has written four books on pet care. His latest book How To Care For Your Pet Bird: Practical Advice From Dr. Joel Murphy just rolled off the presses recently.

Dr. Murphy gives lectures at veterinary continuing education conferences and animal and bird societies yearly. He has published 112 articles and 12 scientific papers. He produced a complete "How To" pet video series in 1988. He has been featured on many radio shows and also on Good Morning America.

**Advanced Training in Veterinary Care for His Clients**

Dr. Murphy graduated Cum Laude from Virginia Tech with a double bachelor's degree in biochemistry and animal psychology. He received his doctorate in veterinary medicine from the world-renowned University of Georgia Veterinary School. He was one of four students out of his entire veterinary class that qualified for an additional year of extremely rigorous training in dog and cat medicine and surgery. This was the most intense year of advanced training as he worked hand in hand with some of the top dermatologists, neurologists, orthopedic surgeons, radiologists and internal medicine specialists in the country. In addition to his advanced training in the diagnosis and treatment of dog and cat diseases, he served as Director of Exotic Animal and Bird Medicine at the University of Georgia Veterinary School and taught all of the exotic animal and bird classes to student veterinarians.

**Holistic Medicine**

In addition to state of the art medicine and surgery performed daily with dogs, cats and all other species,, Dr. Murphy has been studying homeopathy, herbal medicine, flower essences, nutraceuticals, Reiki and adamantine medicine for over 20 years and uses these regularly in treating his diverse group of patients in practice. Dr. Murphy has been well-known across the United States for his holistic supplements that have been sold in quality health food stores by the Renew Life Company in the past. He is now creating extraordinary herbal formulas for Vital Planet Pets.

**The Highest Level of Expertise in Pet Bird Medicine**

He is one of the first veterinarians in the world to become diplomat, American Board of Veterinary Practitioners Certified in Avian Practice. This is the only advanced certification for exotic bird medicine and this level of expertise requires an extremely high level of training and testing. In addition, Dr. Murphy founded the Murphy Exotic Bird Research Center, one of the largest nonprofit bird sanctuaries for the study of how to best care for your parrots. Dr. Murphy has been doing research in the Amazon rainforest for 15 years, studying habitat and natural diets of parrots in the wild. This led to his study of flower essences and the creation of his flower essence company, Rainflower Essence – www.rainfloweressence.com.

# TABLE OF **CONTENTS**

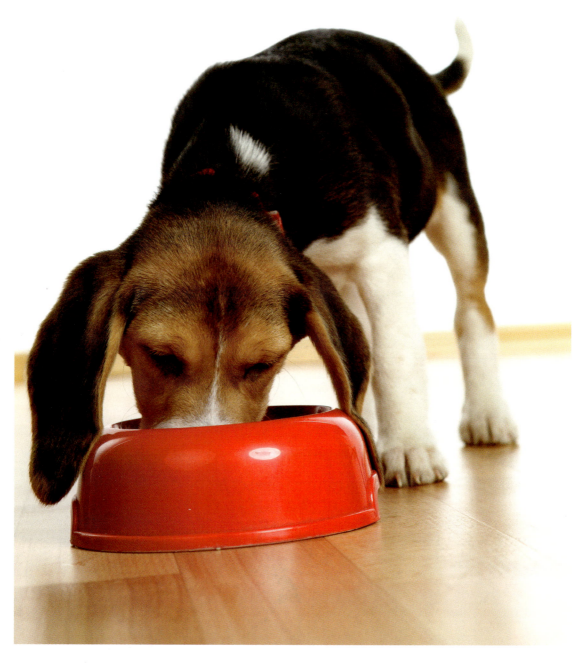

## CHAPTER 1

# THE HEALTHY
# DIGESTIVE SYSTEM

More and more of our canine population seems to suffer from some form of digestive stress. I'm sure you notice when your sweet dog spits up, has bad breath, a change in poop consistency or loss of appetite, or even a bit of a bloated belly. Digestive functions are definitely a good pet parent's primary way to monitor the overall health of your dog. That is why the first thing your veterinarian asks when you bring in your dog "what does his poop look like?"

You may have already heard how important your dog's digestion is to his overall health. Maybe you've surrendered other pups to chronic diseases and this time you just want to know how to be sure your four-legged friend has the best chance to lead a vital and healthy life. Whatever your health goal for your pet, the journey to achieving that goal begins with a clear understanding of a healthy digestive system.

# **MY HEARTFELT** GOALS

- If you are reading this for your puppy, my goal is to help guide you to make the most appropriate choices to nourish, support, and maintain your new pet's optimum health for many, many years to come, taking into consideration your finances and time constraints as well.

- If you are reading this because you just rescued your new best friend, you may have very little idea of their previous health history and now you are in the position to restore wellness on all levels. Rescue organizations have established themselves as guardian angels in the realm of finding and placing dogs in joyful forever homes, however when you receive your dog, he or she may simply have been checked for the basic worm issues and given age appropriate vaccinations. Even a young dog could have been compromised nutritionally. I will suggest ways to insure your pet has the best chance for a healthy and happy life, moving forward.

- If you are reading this for a more mature dog who has been in your home for many years and who may be diagnosed with "age-related diseases" like arthritis, obesity, or kidney or liver stress, my goal is to share with you how to help heal him from the inside out. It is never too late to improve your dog's health. As you implement my easy suggestions, you will have the great joy of seeing your companion move more easily, brighten up and generally become "younger".

Many of my human clients over the last decades while I was teaching about digestive health have told me that one day they realized that they had – for example – arthritis, or 'all of a sudden' they had high blood pressure, and very often one form or another of diabetes.

The concepts of health that I am about to share are true for both yourself and also for your dog. The conditions I mentioned and MANY more have actually been brewing silently for years – in the gut! A little inflammation here, a bit of inflammation there, no symptoms right away – and then one day – it's like the campfire finally catches life – and your doctor diagnoses arthritis, diabetes, heart issues, allergies, the list is a mighty one!

**THE PROCESS IS VERY MUCH THE SAME FOR YOUR DOG OR CAT!**

So let's gain understanding of this process – and understand that Healthy Gut = Healthy Life!

**No wonder your dog's natural response will be bow WOW!!!**

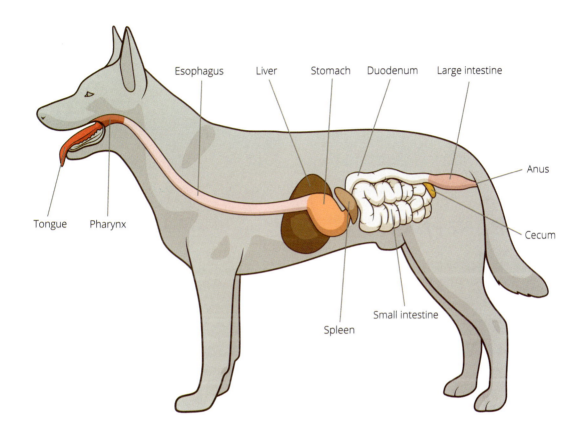

Esophagus · Liver · Stomach · Duodenum · Large intestine · Anus · Cecum · Small intestine · Spleen · Tongue · Pharynx

# WHAT IS DIGESTION?

Digestion encompasses the chemical and motor (physical motion) activities that breaks down food into its most basic components so that they can be absorbed through the lining of the small intestine. In other words, digestion is the process of converting food into chemical substances that can be absorbed and assimilated. It begins in your dog's mouth with the act of slicing or tearing large chunks of food with their jagged teeth and ends in the large intestine or colon.

## What Does the Digestive System Do?

The digestive system has two broad functions: The first and best known is the digestion and absorption of food. The second function is the excretion of wastes. Both of these occur primarily in the small and large intestines. Just as true in dogs as it is in humans is the phrase, "The road to health is paved with good intestines."

## What Organs Make Up the Digestive System?

The digestive tract is a tube roughly four times the length of your dog's body that begins with the mouth and ends with the anus. The digestive system (or gastrointestinal tract) is made up of the mouth, esophagus, stomach, small intestine, large intestine and anus. Along this tube are accessory organs like the teeth, tongue, salivary glands, gallbladder, liver and pancreas.

## What Are the Specific Functions of the Digestive System?

**The digestive tract has three primary functions:**

- **Motor** – assisting food movement
- **Secretory** – preparing food for absorption by producing digestive enzymes
- **Absorptive** – breaking food down and converting food parts into substances that can be absorbed through digestion

## THE DIGESTIVE PROCESS

In dogs, the chemical breakdown of food begins in the stomach. They don't have digestive enzymes in their saliva as we do (in humans, starch digestion begins in the mouth with the enzyme amylase.) However, dog saliva does contain antibacterial chemicals. This explains why your dog will lick her superficial wounds, actually cleaning them. It's also part of the reason why your dog may eat scary, smelly stuff and not get sick!

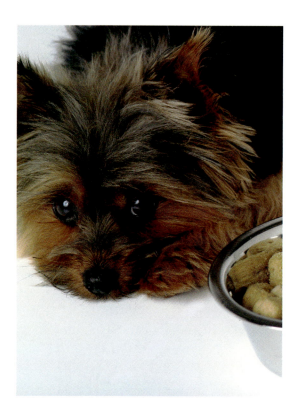

Food is swallowed rapidly and transferred down the esophagus to the stomach. Dogs are designed to ingest large chunks of meat, bones and organs. Since their jaws only move up and down (not sideways) they are not able to chew their food, thus seeming to gulp down their dinners. Remember, in dogs - the first place food really begins to break down is in the stomach.

### The Esophagus

The esophagus is a long muscular tube, lined with mucus-producing cells, which lubricates the food so that it passes through with ease. The esophagus transports food to the stomach through the action of its wave-like muscular contractions (peristalsis). It is coated with a protective mucous lining. The muscular valve at the bottom of the esophagus is known as the lower esophageal sphincter. This valve remains tightly closed when food is not being eaten so that stomach acid cannot back into the esophagus. It opens and closes quickly to allow food to pass into the stomach.

## Peristalsis in the Esophagus

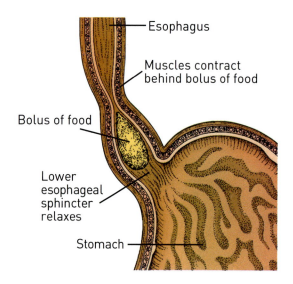

Esophagus

Muscles contract behind bolus of food

Bolus of food

Lower esophageal sphincter relaxes

Stomach

Dogs have a natural regurgitation response. Occasionally they will spit out food and/or liquid from the esophagus that for some reason doesn't pass easily to the stomach. Many times they will then proceed to eat it again! I've wondered about this in the past. Perhaps you have too.

In nature, occasional regurgitation is actually a normal behavior. It happens suddenly and without discomfort. Since in most cases, the food has not reached the stomach it appears similar to when eaten. Generally regurgitated dinner doesn't even smell like vomit.

As a first response, in our sanitary lives, we tend to run to clean up the "mess".

> ## EXPERIMENT:
> Next time your dog spits up, leave it for a bit and see if he eats it again. If he does, he has regurgitated his food.

**Important point** – regurgitation is different from vomiting. Where regurgitation is a passive process involving the esophagus, vomiting is a forceful active process, ejecting the stomach or sometimes the intestinal contents. Vomit will often have a foul smell arising from the partially digested food, mucus and possible intestinal liquids.

**If either vomiting or regurgitation occurs very often, consult your veterinarian.**

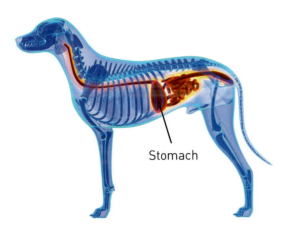

Stomach

 **TIP** Videotaping the occurrence can be helpful for the doctor to differentiate regurgitation (an esophageal process) from vomiting which can indicate many disease processes.

## The Stomach

As you now know, in dogs, chemical breakdown of food begins in the mouth, specifically the breakdown of protein.

The dog's stomach pH is extremely low with a pH of 1-2 due to his high concentration of hydrochloric acid (HCl) and enzymes. Your dog's healthy stomach is much more acidic than yours. This extreme acidity ensures an efficient breakdown of meat and bones and protects your dog from bad bacteria and microbes.

A mucous lining coats the cells of the stomach to protect them from the HCl and enzymes that must be present for proper digestion. Damage to this lining can often lead to gastritis (irritation of the stomach lining) just as in humans.

**Hydrochloric acid** (HCl) is produced by parietal cells (tiny pumps) in the lining of the stomach. This acid is needed to ensure the proper functioning of the stomach.

> **HCl has two primary functions:**
> - It provides the acidic environment necessary for the enzyme pepsin to break down proteins
> - It helps prevent infection by destroying most parasites and bacteria

At the end of the stomach is the pyloric sphincter, which controls the opening between the end of the stomach and the duodenum which is the first section of the small intestine.

## The Duodenum

When food leaves the stomach, it enters the first section of the small intestine-the duodenum. The mixture is now called chyme, a mixture of food, HCl and mucus, which is approximately the consistency of split pea soup.

**As the duodenum fills, hormones released from the duodenal lining:**

- Delay emptying of the stomach
- Promote bile flow from the liver and gallbladder
- Promote secretion of water, bicarbonate and potent digestive enzymes from the pancreas

The surface of the duodenum is smooth for the first few inches, but quickly changes to a surface with many folds and small finger-like projections called villi or microvilli (very small projections). These projections serve to increase the surface area and absorption capabilities of the duodenum.

Properly functioning accessory organs (liver, gallbladder and pancreas) are crucial during this first-stage of digestion.

## Pancreas

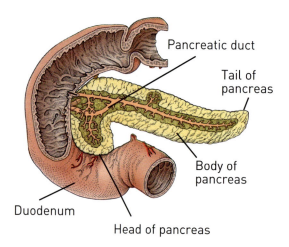

Pancreatic duct

Tail of pancreas

Body of pancreas

Duodenum

Head of pancreas

## The Pancreas

**The pancreas has three main functions important to a dog's digestion:**

- Neutralizes stomach acid
- Regulates blood sugar levels
- Produces digestive enzymes

Digestive enzymes digest proteins, carbohydrates and fats. These secretions (pancreatic enzymes and bicarbonates) are delivered directly into the duodenum, the upper portion of the small intestine. The pancreas also secretes hormones which help manage blood sugar levels, directly into the bloodstream. These hormones are insulin (sugar lowering) and glucagon (sugar raising). High percentages of carbohydrates in your dog's diet puts a lot of stress on pancreatic function.

## The Liver and Gallbladder

The liver has several important functions, a number of which are related to digestion. It performs over 1000 important tasks that cannot be done elsewhere in the body.

**The liver:**

- Functions as your dog's primary organ of detoxification
- Produces albumin, the main protein in blood
- Produces bile from cholesterol
- Stores fat-soluble vitamins such as A, D, E and K
- Produces blood clotting factors
- Stores energy

And these are only a few of the liver's important functions. About 80% of the cholesterol produced by the liver is used to make bile, which is critical in proper digestion of fat. Bile is composed of bile salts, hormones (including cholesterol) and toxins. It acts to blend and distribute fat, cholesterol and fat soluble vitamins throughout the intestines. Bile, an alkaline substance, also neutralizes stomach acid. Between meals, it is stored in the gallbladder, a pear-shaped organ located just below the liver. When liquidified food (chyme) enters the duodenum, a signal is sent to the gallbladder to contract, thereby releasing bile into the duodenum.

The liver is remarkable in another important way. It has the unique ability to regenerate itself under certain circumstances! It can recover both tissue and functionality when necessary.

The liver functions tirelessly 24/7, carrying out its functions through the bloodstream. Every blood vessel leaving the gastrointestinal tract goes directly to the liver, and the liver is the first tissue to receive and process the nutrients absorbed by the intestines.

A complete discussion of the amazing functions of the liver (in both dogs and humans) is beyond the scope of this book. Suffice it to say, a healthy liver is a strong assurance of health and vitality!

## The Small Intestine

> **The entire small intestine consists of three sections:**
>
> • **The duodenum** – primarily absorbs minerals
>
> • **The jejunum** – absorbs water-soluble vitamins, carbohydrates and proteins
>
> • **The ileum** – absorbs fat soluble vitamins, fat, cholesterol and bile salts.

The walls of the small intestine secrete alkaline digestive enzymes, which continue the separation of foods—proteins into amino acids, fats into fatty acids and glycerin and carbohydrates into simple sugars.

# Intestinal Cross-section

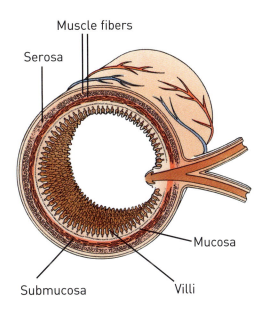

Muscle fibers

Serosa

Mucosa

Submucosa

Villi

Ninety percent of all nutrients are absorbed in the small intestine, which can be considered your dog's major digestive organ. The small intestine resembles a coiled hose. It is here that most food completes the digestion process.

> **The small intestine contains cells that serve many functions:**
>
> • Some produce mucus
>
> • Some make enzymes
>
> • Some absorb nutrients
>
> • Others are capable of killing bad bacteria and other microbes

As discussed previously, the cells are arranged in folds upon folds, which force the chyme to move slower, so it can be broken down completely and absorbed. These folds also increase the surface area of the mucosa, the thin mucous membrane lining the walls of the entire small intestine.

# THERE IS A SAYING "YOU ARE WHAT YOU EAT". I WOULD LIKE TO SHIFT THAT TO "YOU ARE WHAT YOU ABSORB"! YOUR GOOD HEALTH IS TOTALLY DEPENDENT ON YOUR DIGESTIVE CAPABILITIES.

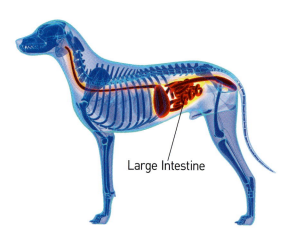

Large Intestine

## The Colon or Large Intestine

The last organ through which food residue passes is the colon or large intestine. The large intestine participates in the last phase of digestion, performing three very important functions.

- It recovers the last available water and electrolytes from the food consumed
- It forms and stores feces
- It works with bacteria to produce enzymes capable of breaking down difficult-to-digest material.

The colon is the largest part of the large intestine and the terms are often used interchangeably. Chyme enters the large intestine through the ileocecal valve (ICV), a one-way valve that connects the small and large intestines. This valve regulates the flow of chyme entering the large intestine.

The ICV is designed to let waste pass into the large intestine and prevent it from backing into the small intestine. At this juncture, chyme is still

in a liquid state. The cecum is the first section of the large intestine. Food waste travels through rhythmic waves of contraction (peristalsis) through the large intestine. As it moves, the liquid is extracted.

## THE PRIMARY JOB OF THE COLON IS TO ABSORB WATER AND ELECTROLYTES FROM THE CHYME, FORMING FECES.

The fecal matter is in a semi solid state, gradually becoming firmer, as it continues through the colon. About two-thirds of stool is water, undigested fiber and food products; one-third is living and dead bacteria (bacteria naturally live in the colon). As you will learn, good bacterial balance in the intestinal tract is critical for proper digestion, overall well-being and healthy bowel movements in your dog.

**The large intestine also:**

- Secretes bicarbonate to neutralize acid end products
- Stores waste products, bacteria and intestinal gas
- Excretes poisons and waste products from the body

The rectum is the chamber at the end of the large intestine. Fecal matter passes into the rectum, creating the urge to defecate. The anus is the opening at the far end of the digestive tract. The anus allows fecal matter to pass out of the body. The anal sphincters keep the anus closed.

Your dog has two anal sacs, also called anal glands, located on the lower sides of his anus. They produce an excretion with a scent that identifies him and tells other dogs such things as your dog's sex, health and approximate age. These sacs excrete this fluid when the dog has a bowel movement. These glands can become impacted and cause health issues through lack of appropriate dietary fiber.

## The Mucous Membrane

The walls of both the small and large intestines consist of four layers. The innermost layer of the small intestine is called the mucosa.

**The mucosa has two very important functions:**

- It is designed to allow nutrients of the proper size to pass through it and into the bloodstream.
- The mucosa blocks the passage of undigested food particles, parasites, bacteria and toxins into the bloodstream.

Therefore, the mucosa or mucosal lining is a vital part of the dog's immune system because it limits the volume of potential invaders.

## 80% OF A DOG'S IMMUNE SYSTEM IS IN THE **DIGESTIVE SYSTEM.**

As you've learned, the mucosa is lined with villi and microvilli. The villi are moving absorptive cells that "suck up" small particles of digested food. On each of the villi are thousands of tiny projections of the membrane of the cell called microvilli. These little brush-like fuzzy structures (called the "brush border") further amplify the surface area of the small intestine.

On the surface of this mucosal lining is a thick mucous layer whose surface is highly viscous (slippery).Much of the mucus consists of the amino sugar N-acetyl-glucosamine (NAG). The body makes NAG from the amino acid L-glutamine. L-glutamine exists in virtually all cells, and it is one of the most prevalent amino acids in the body.

## DOGS MUST HAVE L-GLUTAMINE IN ORDER TO PRODUCE NAG AND HAVE A HEALTHY MUCOSAL LINING.

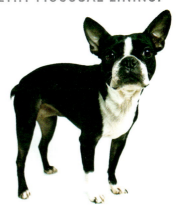

The mucosal lining in a healthy intestine sheds, and then is rebuilt every three to five days. Studies have shown that dogs suffering from any inflammatory bowel disease shed this mucosal layer at a much higher rate. This may be due to an inability to convert L-glutamine into NAG.

## The Immune System in the Gut

The gut is the largest immune organ in the body as its job is to allow absorption of food, while excluding elements like harmful bacteria and toxins. It is the main route of contact with the external environment. Think of it like the skin – only on the inside of the body.

The intestinal tract is bombarded with food, toxins and microbes. Somehow, your dog's body is able to examine this mess and decide which of the substances he ingests are good and which ones are bad.

The immune system of the digestive tract has a huge responsibility in maintaining health – every bite of food that a dog eats has hundreds to thousands of different proteins that the immune system has to check and determine if these proteins are safe or toxic.

This is why the digestive system is your dog's biggest ally in immunity.

## DR. MURPHY

The GI system is overloaded every day with external stimuli. On a daily basis, beneficial substances (like food) and unthreatening microbes in the environment enter your dog's body. Additionally, your dog's intestinal tract is regularly confronted with potentially dangerous pathogenic microbes (bacteria, protozoa, fungi, viruses) and/or various toxic substances.

The crucial position of the gastrointestinal system is testified by the huge amount of immune cells that reside within it. Indeed, gut-associated lymphoid tissue (GALT) is the prominent part of mucosal-associated lymphoid tissue (MALT) and represents almost 70% of the entire immune system; moreover, about 80% of plasma cells [mainly immunoglobulin A (IgA)-bearing cells] reside in the GALT. The immune mechanisms functioning in the GI tract are extremely complex and beyond the scope of this book. Suffice it to say, since the stomach, intestines and colon come in direct contact with the external environment, the GI system must protect your dog from dangerous substances potentially entering the bloodstream of his body through the mucosal lining.

An important thing to understand is that health in the digestive tract is maintained by the constant sensing and scanning performed by the cells of the immune system. It is an active function and not just a situation of the immune cells ignoring certain things. The immune system is actually a tricky balance between a pro-inflammatory response and an anti-inflammatory one.

If this balance is not maintained, the immune system can become over-reactive to harmless substances (as in the case of allergies and sensitivities) and lead to inflammatory disease. On the other hand, if the immune system becomes overly anti-inflammatory, dangerous pathogens would not be kept under control.

**THE GI SYSTEM** IS WHERE BACTERIA AND OTHER MICROBES ALONG WITH VARIOUS SUBSTANCES, BOTH BENEFICIAL AND HARMFUL, MEET YOUR DOG.

### The Digestive Environment

It is difficult to fully understand the digestive system without realizing the importance of the bacteria and microbes that live in your dog's intestinal tract.

**Good bacteria:**

- Provide immunity through inhibiting bad bacteria
- Make vitamins
- Ferment fiber for good bowel movements
- Breakdown toxins
- Repair intestinal walls
- Provide many other functions as your dog grows and matures

A new-born puppy has essentially no digestive bacteria. Within a few hours, the bacteria and microbes begin to colonize the digestive tract through the antibody loaded first milk produced

## Healthy Digestive Tract

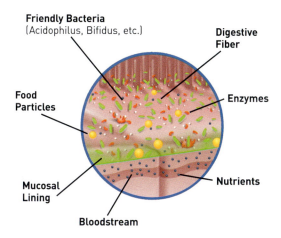

Friendly Bacteria
(Acidophilus, Bifidus, etc.)

Digestive Fiber

Food Particles

Enzymes

Mucosal Lining

Nutrients

Bloodstream

Once the puppy's digestive system begins to mature, the bacterial balance in the digestive system will largely be determined by diet and genetics. A healthy diet will promote beneficial fermentation processes in the intestines, create an environment for good bacteria and will help to sustain a resilient mucous lining, important for both immunity and absorption of proper nutrients.

Bad bacteria produce substances that are harmful to the body. They irritate the lining of the intestines (causing gas) and can be absorbed into the bloodstream (causing disease). They cannot always be prevented from entering the body, but if the number of good and neutral bacteria stays high, then, theoretically, the bad bacteria will be kept to a minimum.

The neutral bacteria are the most prevalent bacteria in the digestive tract. Neutral microbes have neither a positive nor negative impact. As your dog ages, the levels of bad bacteria tend to increase, and relatively the good bacteria decrease. We will further clarify this important point in future chapters.

by the mother. This is called colostrum, which is defined as the first 24-48 hours of milk following birth. This colostrum contains highly concentrated large protein antibody molecules, water, vitamins, electrolytes and nutrients.

Many breeders and dog owners assume that a puppy is receiving antibodies as long as they are nursing. This is simply not the case. Newborn puppies lose their ability to absorb these antibodies at approximately 18 hours after birth. As in human babies, nursing immediately ensures the best possibility of promoting a healthy digestive environment throughout the newborn dog's life.

Additionally, the health and immunity of the mother determines the amount of antibodies that she has to pass to her babes via colostrum. This is known as antibody titer. It is a good idea to measure the mother's titer before breeding since a healthy mother will be able to pass along more protection to her young. The babies will then possess higher levels of protection for longer periods of time against the diseases that the mother has immunity against such as canine distemper, canine parvovirus and canine coronavirus.

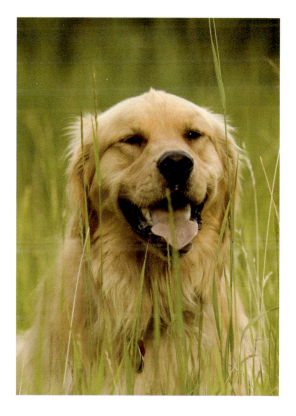

## The Signs of Good Digestion and Elimination

Dogs have the shortest digestive systems of mammals. It takes roughly 8-9 hours for complete digestion of food in a healthy dog.

At a minimum, your dog should have one good bowel movement per day, but two to three are not unusual. Check your dog's stool for color and consistency. A "normal" movement will be chocolate brown in color, with a consistency a bit like putty when pressed, formed into a somewhat oblong shape. When you pick it up in the doggy bag, it should be a bit soft, however retain its form without melting into the grass.

Hard stool could indicate dehydration. Loose stool might point to the large intestine not re-absorbing water and could be caused by something irritating your dog's gut that she thought was delicious. Loose stool can also indicate many other issues.

Since dogs can't directly talk to us, their stool is used frequently to determine what internal

processes may be out of balance. And many stool issues can and will occur. So we, as concerned pet parents must become avid poop peepers!

Fortunately, many poop issues in dogs resolve on their own within 24 hours. If an unusual color of stool (black, red streaks, gray or yellow) or unusual consistency persists, it's time to ring up your veterinarian as unusual stool may indicate a serious issue.

THE REASON MOST OF THE IMMUNE SYSTEM IS IN THE DIGESTIVE TRACT IS THAT **MOST OF THE BODY'S CONTACT WITH TOXINS AND UNHEALTHY BACTERIA OCCUR IN THE INTESTINAL TRACT,** WHICH OVER TIME, CAUSES DISEASE IN DOGS.

## Ideal Elimination Cycle

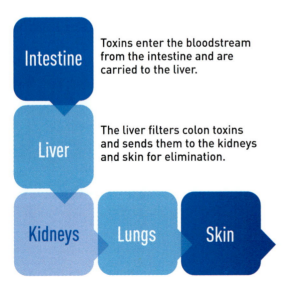

**Intestine** — Toxins enter the bloodstream from the intestine and are carried to the liver.

**Liver** — The liver filters colon toxins and sends them to the kidneys and skin for elimination.

**Kidneys** **Lungs** **Skin**

**PROPER FUNCTION OF THE SEVEN CHANNELS OF ELIMINATION = HEALTHY DETOXIFICATION = VIBRANT LIFE!**

The seven channels of elimination are:
- **Colon**
- **Lungs**
- **Liver**
- **Skin**
- **Kidneys**
- **Blood**
- **Lymph**

The first five of these channels are all organs. We've just taken a basic look at how your colon and liver aid in the process of detoxification. The blood that flows through the vessels of the vascular (blood circulatory) system carries oxygen and nutrients to the cells of the body

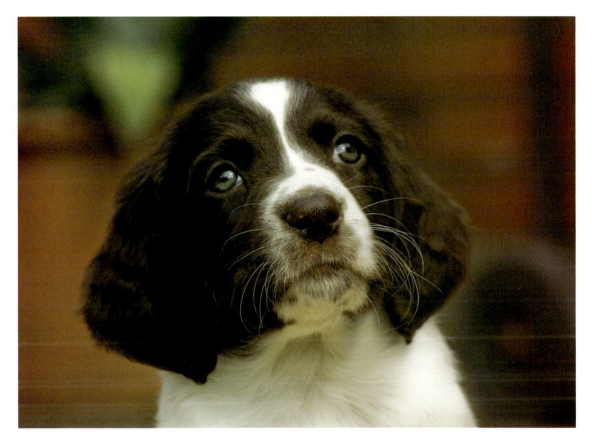

YOUR DOG'S LYMPH NODES ARE CONCENTRATED IN THE GROIN, UNDER YOUR DOG'S FRONT LEGS, IN THE NECK AND ABDOMEN; THEY FILTER LYMPH AND PRODUCE LYMPHOCYTES.

and removes harmful wastes. Not so familiar to many is the other circulatory system, the lymphatic system, through which lymph flows.

## The Lymph

The lymphatic system and the vascular system work together to eliminate poisons from cells. The lymphatic system consists of a network of vessels that extends throughout your dog's body, following the path of the veins. The lymphatic capillaries contain a clear fluid—lymph—which carries lymphocytes (immune cells). The lymphatic system is an important part of the immune system. In fact, organs of the immune system are known as "lymphoid organs."

**They include the following:**

- **Bone marrow -** Where white blood cells originate

- **Spleen -** A filter for the lymphatic system and a storage site for white blood cells.

- **Liver -** The major detoxification organ of your dog's body

- **Lymph nodes -** Small bean shaped structures that connect with lymphatic capillaries

- **Thymus gland** – Home of the T cells, which mobilize the body's defense system when the immune system is challenged

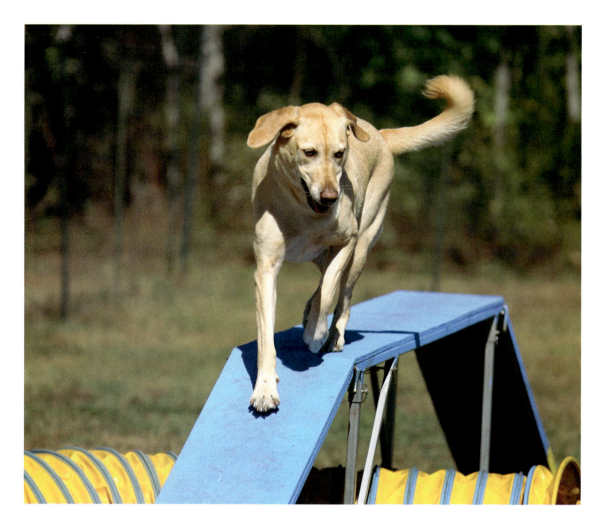

All these lymphoid organs are concerned with the growth, development and deployment of white blood cells (lymphocytes), whose function it is to defend the body against antigens (substances the body perceives as foreign and threatening, such as viruses, fungi, bacteria, parasites and pollen).

Healthy lymph nodes are small structures, barely detectable, most often less than ½ inch in diameter (depending on your dog's breed). Don't be concerned if you can't feel them easily. That's a good thing which means they're functioning properly and are not swollen.

It's a great idea to familiarize yourself with the location of your dog's lymph nodes so you'll recognize any change. They can most easily be located by gently feeling under the lower jaw where it connects with the neck area, the front part of the shoulder area, by the back of the thigh, by the armpit, and by the groin where the thigh connects with the abdomen. If you notice unusual swelling or hardness, consider a visit to your vet.

## The Kidneys

The kidneys are two bean-shaped organs located just under your dog's diaphragm in the back. The liver sends water-soluble wastes to the kidneys via the blood where this waste is eliminated through the bladder.

The kidneys are considered the "great purifiers" of the body. The kidneys determine which chemicals

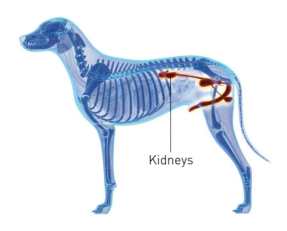

Kidneys

are needed by the body, absorb them and filter out the rest. The kidneys have the additional function of maintaining water balance.

Healthy kidneys depend on making absolutely certain your dog has adequate hydration all the time, both through her food as well as a clean and available fresh water source.

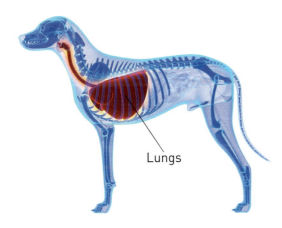

Lungs

## The Lungs

The lungs, another secondary elimination organ, expel toxins from the body. One of the most common toxins is carbon dioxide. The action of breathing helps to move lymph and blood through the body, and with it, toxins.

The lungs are lined with mucus and cilia (hair-like projections) to help protect against and remove inhaled toxins and are normally coughed

up or swallowed. Many microorganisms live in the normally healthy respiratory system. The balance of good to bad bacteria is held in check by local and systemic immune factors.

Normal respiratory rates vary from 10 to 30 breaths per minute depending on the size of your dog; larger dogs have slower rates. Panting a rapid, open-mouthed, and shallow breathing pattern is a normal behavior, stimulated by exercise and/or the need to cool the body.

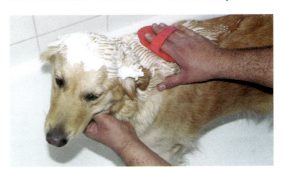

## The Skin

A dog's skin and coat are a reflection of the internal health of your pet and therefore a very important indicator of his health. When a dog is healthy internally, the body's normal metabolic processes provide the hair follicles with all the of the nutrients needed to have a lustrous coat.

**The skin is the largest organ in a dog's body. Your dog's skin and fur:**

- Provide a barrier against bacteria, viruses and fungal infections
- Protect the dog's internal organs
- "Breathe" and are an important organ of detoxification
- Critical to maintaining a balanced body temperature
- Prevent dehydration
- Provide sensory information about the surrounding environment

A healthy skin and coat are strong indicators of a healthy and happy dog.

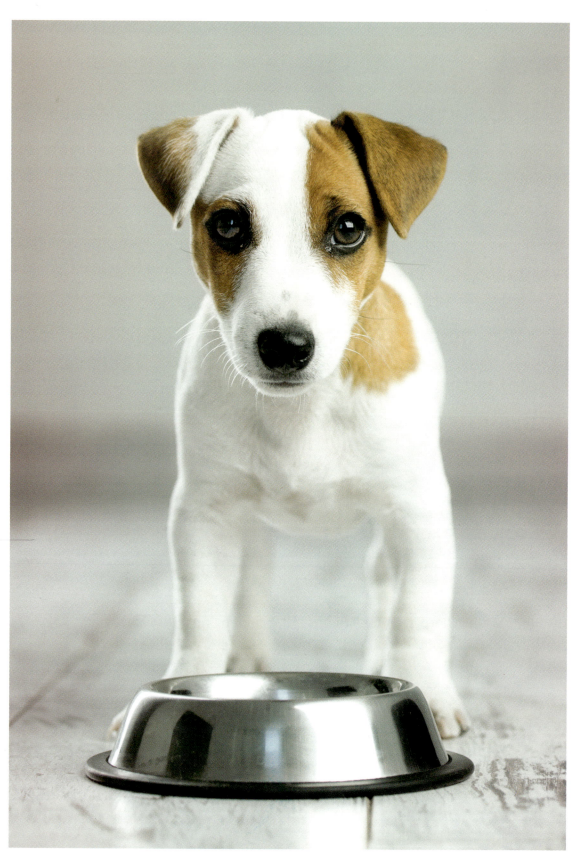

# CHAPTER 2

# IMPAIRED
# **DIGESTION**

At this point I'd like you to take a look with me at the process of declining health that happens to many dogs. Poor health actually begins in the digestive system, which is why my passionate message has been for so many years – first for humans and now for dogs – "All health begins in the gut".

Impaired digestion is the beginning of a process that ends with chronic disease, in both people and their pets (see figure 1). Throughout life, there are many factors that can and do influence the process. Some of the factors that impact our pets' digestion are diet, genetics, environmental toxins, pharmaceutical medications and even stress. The only one not controlled easily by an educated pet parent is genetics. A closer look at the digestive system reveals the effects of these influences.

Canine vomiting and diarrhea are the most common complaints that veterinarians treat. Part of this is the nature of the dog. Dogs tend to eat everything they find that has an appealing smell or taste. As we touched on in the previous chapter, the canine digestive system is designed to reject (by spitting up) anything that upsets the delicate lining of the esophagus, stomach and digestive tract. The fact that dogs (and cats) vomit much easier than people is actually their first defense against ingesting toxic compounds. The dog's saliva, which you learned contains antibacterial chemicals along with the acids in dogs' stomachs are designed to sterilize the food they eat by killing most of the bacteria and fungi that they ingest. The digestive system, along with absorbing nutrients and water from the food dogs eat also functions as one of the most important methods of eliminating waste and toxins from the body.

# DR. MURPHY

It is important for pet owners to realize that vomiting and diarrhea can be the symptom of a mild problem or symptom of serious disease. Monitor your pet for frequency and severity of vomiting and diarrhea and consult with your veterinarian. This, along with a thorough physical exam, will help your veterinarian determine how intensive a diagnostic workup is indicated when your dog has vomiting or diarrhea. As you can see from the list below diagnosing the cause of vomiting and diarrhea in dogs requires a lot of training, diagnostic tests and decision making.

**Just a few Causes of Vomiting and Diarrhea:**

- Eating too fast
- Change in food from one brand to another
- Parasites such as hookworms, whip worms, Giardia, coccidia, Physaloptera and round worms
- Toxic people medications such as aspirin, ibuprofen, Tylenol
- Toxic chemicals such as home insecticides, antifreeze, rat poison, even the plant - lilies

- Toxic human foods such a xylitol, grapes, raisins, macadamia nuts
- Bacterial infections of the gastrointestinal tract such as E.coli,Campylobacter, Clostridium and Salmonella
- Bacterial toxins – eating garbage and dead wildlife, frogs, lizards
- Viral diseases such as distemper, parvovirus, coronavirus, rotavirus
- Dietary protein intolerance – protein allergies
- Side effect of medications such as antibiotics
- Hemorrhagic gastroenteritis
- Addison's disease
- Diabetes mellitus and ketoacidosis
- Kidney failure
- Liver disease
- Pancreatitis
- Inflammatory bowel disease
- Head trauma
- Protein-losing enteropathy
- Stomach torsion and volvulus
- Obstruction by foreign bodies such as toys, plastic, towels, socks
- Cancer

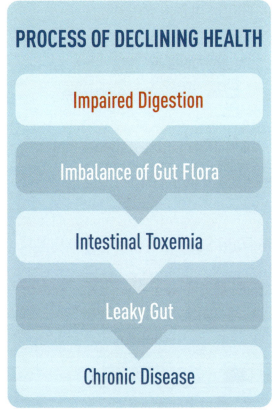

## PROCESS OF DECLINING HEALTH

Impaired Digestion

Imbalance of Gut Flora

Intestinal Toxemia

Leaky Gut

Chronic Disease

(Figure 1)

It's important for you to realize that just about every disease a pet may contract either begins with or ultimately affects the delicate lining of the digestive tract and often triggers a bout of vomiting and/or diarrhea. Therefore awareness of the frequency and consistency of spitting up and/or uncommon bowel movements can help you differentiate between normal regurgitation and poop and the possibility of an underlying disease process in the making.

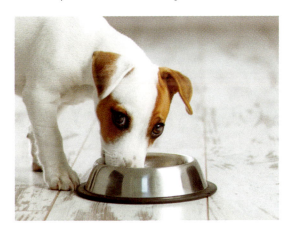

**Many of the issues that result in impaired digestion may be part of your dog's daily life that you could positively influence:**

- Processed food consumption, both regular food and treats
- Overeating
- Stress
- Mental / Emotional
- Physical
- Viral
- Chemical and Environmental
- Lowered production of enzymes
- Imbalanced intestinal pH

Sadly, any of the above factors, alone or most often in conjunction with the others, inevitably can lead to weight issues or various other less obvious internal problems. The following section explores these causative factors in more detail.

## CAUSES OF IMPAIRED DIGESTION

### Processed Food Consumption

Processed dog foods such as canned food and kibble are those that have been through a commercial refining process, which includes the application of high temperatures. Such processing serves the purpose of increasing shelf life. The down side is that it also destroys life supporting nutrients, creating a situation of imbalance and deficiency.

The diagrams presented above demonstrate how dog food is made. The top diagram represents canned, wet dog food, and the bottom shows the process taken to create kibble.

## A PROCESS COMMONLY USED TO CREATE DOG FOOD SOLD IN A CAN (WET)

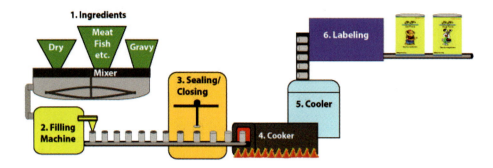

## A PROCESS COMMONLY USED TO CREATE DOG FOOD SOLD IN A BAG (DRY/KIBBLE)

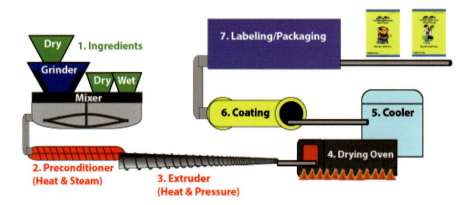

Both of these diagrams have one disturbing step in common. Please notice #4 in both. As you learned above, applying heat to foods completely eliminates any living components within the food. Once in a can or bag, the food you buy from the grocery store is essentially dead food. Pet owners don't realize this and a large number of dogs eat dead food a great majority of the time.

You may be wondering, what living essential components are being killed? Isn't it a good idea to sterilize food to remove bad bacteria and possible germs?

There are three critical components of healthful food that are ruined when heated. Enzymes, probiotics and omega oils. We will discuss their importance in greater detail as our story continues.

Additionally, there is much conversation currently regarding a "species appropriate" diet for dogs. This refers to the understanding that dogs are carnivores. From this perspective, carbohydrates (grains, starchy vegetables) are unnecessary for your dog's well-being and in fact stress the digestive process.

We have seen sugar and carbohydrates distort the bodies of the American population since the 1960's. Sadly, the same has been happening to our pets. When grains are milled into flour, the starch they contain becomes a high-glycemic (more sugary) food and can cause obesity in both you and your pets.

There is much varying opinion about proper feeding of our dogs. I will be sharing some insights into feeding in an upcoming chapter of this book with you. I promise to offer you many options so there will be one that will best suit your financial and time needs and be most nutritionally appropriate for your best friend.

**At this point I'd just like to offer some information about the state of dog food as it is generally available today**.

When dogs lived on farms and ranches across the US, they were generally fed table scraps and what they could scavenge from around the barn. It was rare to see an obese dog. Currently in our country, I was astounded to read that at least 50% of our dogs are considered obese! I believe that statistic requires a closer look into the causes of that health threatening situation.

Initially dog food was meat based, but with the advent of rationing during WWII, grains were cheaper and easier to store for longer periods of time, so they were introduced into the dog's diet. As I mentioned earlier, milled grains turn a previously protein rich food into a high-glycemic load food due to the starch they contain.

For cows, goats and chickens, grain is an appropriate daily diet. They are herbivores, with chickens enjoying bugs as well. Dogs are considered primarily carnivores and optimally thrive on diets that are meat (protein) based, derived from fresh whole prey. In the wild, dogs usually consume the abdominal contents of their prey, including organ meats and the pancreas, as contrasted with other pure carnivores such as cats that prefer the skeletal muscle and bone. This offers the wild dog a wide variety of nutrients for their health.

Being a carnivore with limited omnivorous (eating both plants and animals) ability, your dog is designed to digest only small amounts of carbohydrates in her diet. Emphasis on "small amounts". And of course, I'm totally aware that your dog won't be out catching her prey for dinner. With regard to your dog's diet, I believe it's important to find a middle ground. Fortunately, your dog is adaptable, and remarkably resilient!

**Bottom line** - Dead food along with excess carbohydrates that your dog doesn't need are key offenders in creating impaired digestion. As a species, carbohydrates are a very secondary aspect of a dog's normal diet, thus their bodies just aren't designed to digest a large amount of carbs efficiently.

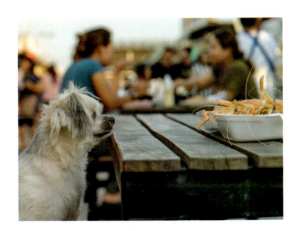

**IMAGINE IF WE ATE CANNED RAVIOLI OR DRY CEREAL EVERY MEAL, EVERY DAY FOR OUR ENTIRE LIFE.**

HOW HEALTHY DO YOU THINK WE'D BE?

## Overeating

As with all of us, chronic overeating ultimately leads to those extra pounds, and obesity. Much of the time it's up to the responsible pet parent to monitor your dog's eating habits and provide the amounts and type of food that keeps your dog in his healthy zone. This is not always an easy task but well worth the effort.

**Here are some conditions that commonly accompany the accumulation of extra pounds on your dog**

- Osteoarthritis and joint issues
- Orthopedic issues
- Type 2 diabetes
- Kidney Disease
- Various skin disorders
- High blood pressure often discovered along with other conditions
- Decreased life expectancy and loss of vitality (can be up to 2.5 years)
- Thyroid problems
- Seizures
- Heart and Respiratory Disease
- Some cancers

**ONE OF THE COMMON PROBLEMS WITH DOG TREATS WHICH CONTRIBUTES TO OBESITY IS THAT THE MAJORITY OF THEM ARE CARBOHYDRATE (STARCH) BASED.** CARBOHYDRATE DIETS CAUSE YOUR DOG'S BODY TO RELEASE LARGE LEVELS OF INSULIN, WHICH JUST LIKE IN PEOPLE, CREATES A COMPLEX OF SYMPTOMS RESULTING IN OBESITY AND INFLAMMATION.

# DR. MURPHY

It's very important to differentiate a bit of bloat caused by overeating from a serious condition known as GDV (Gastric Dilatation and Volvulus) - commonly known as stomach torsion or twisted stomach. Stomach torsion can be life threatening.

Stomach torsion is an especially dangerous cause of vomiting or retching in dogs. It occurs when, due to abnormal peristalsis (the muscle contractions that move food through the intestines), the stomach flips over and cuts off the blood supply to the stomach and spleen. Although it may occur in any breed, stomach torsion is most common in dogs with deep, narrow chests such as Great Danes, Doberman Pinschers, Labrador Retrievers, Golden Retrievers and Bloodhounds.

**Signs of stomach torsion include:**

- Non-productive retching
- Progressive abdominal distension
- Weakness or collapse
- Frequent belching

This is a serious emergency situation, and should this occur, go directly to your local veterinarian. As serious as a person having a heart attack. Any delay in treatment will be fatal. If the stomach cannot be deflated with stomach tubes, immediate surgery is necessary. Most veterinarians will stop everything, cancel or delay current appointments and rush their patient into surgery. If the stomach is returned to normal position within 10-20 minutes, most dogs do well and are discharged in 24 to 72 hours. If the stomach and spleen lose their blood supply for too long, the prognosis is very grave, even with extensive surgery and weeks of hospitalization.

## A PROPER DIET COMBINED WITH SUPPORTIVE SUPPLEMENTATION MAY HELP BRING WEIGHT DOWN – OR KEEP IT WITHIN NORMAL RANGES IN THE FIRST PLACE!

Considering the length of this list and the severity of the potential conditions, it just makes sense to learn all you can about ways to keep your dog within a healthy weight, feeling energetic and living to his full potential. My goal is to help you decrease the stress that too much food puts on the digestive tract.

Along with the health problems that occur with an obese dog, the sheer excess of food puts additional stress on the entire digestive process.

I'm sure you're beginning to realize how extremely important proper digestive health is to the overall health of your dog.

### The Role of Stressors

An often-overlooked reason why our dog's body may fail to digest food properly is stress. Yes, dogs are affected by many different types of stress too! Even though it may seem to you that your dog leads a perfect uncomplicated life, dogs perceive and assimilate the world differently than we humans do.

### Mental and Emotional Stressors

Dog behavior is of great importance to dog owners. A healthy, loving and nurturing emotional bond between humans and pets is what every pet owner wants and deserves. No matter how many human relationships you have, no person will give the unconditional love all the time quite like your dog.

Mental and emotional stress in your dog's life can be as subtle as exposure to new items or people in the house, or as obvious as moving to

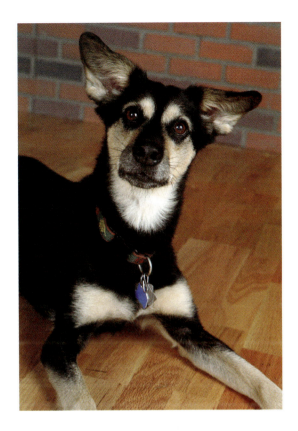

a new home, thunderstorms, or being boarded at a kennel. Whatever the mental/emotional stress, it can have an effect on your dog's digestive system, just as stress can affect your digestion. Here's how:

All unconscious activity in the body is controlled by the autonomic nervous system. The autonomic nervous system controls the digestive system and reactions to stress. Your dog's body is designed to divert energy, blood, enzymes and oxygen away from the digestive organs when stress is experienced. In the wild this would be when your dog would be fleeing from an enemy.

When your dog is under stress, his body releases an excessive amount of a hormone called norephinephrine, which is the "fight or flight" hormone. Norepinephrine directs your dog's body to be ready to run and hide, rather than spend available energy on digesting food. Stress actually lowers the enzyme and acid production that is essential for proper digestion.

From an experiential perspective, before you know it, here comes doggy diarrhea! This increases everyone's stress level, especially if your pet has an accident in the house. You see here just one example of how stress can affect your dog's gut wellness.

I've focused on mental and emotional stressors here, however stress responses can also be triggered by physical and chemical stressors as well, as you will see.

**Triggers that cause stress and anxiety behaviors:**

- Loud noises like thunder, fireworks and construction
- Boarding and kennels
- Veterinary visits
- New pets or family members
- Pet owner phobias
- Training techniques using negative reinforcement

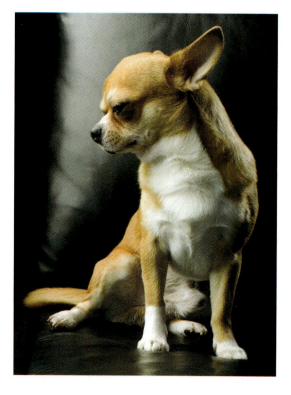

## Physical Stressors

Physical stress is tangible. Infections of all types (even low-grade, sub-clinical ones), as well as trauma from injuries and surgery, are a few examples of physical stress. Dietary indiscretions (such as your pet eating garbage, table scraps, decaying "goodies" your dog discovered outside on a walk) constitute another type of physical stress that can have an adverse effect on her digestive system. The difficult thing about recognizing "stress" is that it subtly increases. It is cumulative over time. It builds quietly until all at once it seems there is a tipping point and your dog may exhibit distressing physical symptoms.

## Viral Stressors

Viral diseases such as distemper, adenovirus and parvovirus cause severe changes and long-term damage to the intestinal tract, mucosa or lining of the intestinal tract and pancreas. These viral diseases are easily and quickly transmitted from dog to dog. The only 100% prevention is keeping your dog away from all contact with other dogs and keeping them away from all the places dogs go. Grass, common neighborhood areas, parks, groomers, day care, training classes, veterinary hospitals. To be truly safe, your pet would need to always be kept indoors. Of course, this is not possible, advisable or enjoyable in most situations for you or your dog!

When this is not appropriate, vaccines are the only way known to holistic and traditional veterinary medicine to successfully prevent these diseases. Veterinary vaccines are time-tested and are proven to work very effectively.

While vaccines will not stress or kill your dog like the viral diseases mentioned, the medicine itself may have a stressful effect on your pet. It's important to work with your veterinarian to determine which vaccines are absolutely necessary. Using diagnostic tools such as vaccine

## DR. MURPHY

Please understand, it is not that veterinarians are not focused on preventative care for pets. Veterinarians are by training already laser focused on preventative care. They understand the health benefits, as well as the cost effectiveness, in preventing rather than treating disease. For example, preventing a parvovirus infection with a simple vaccination costs around $50. Treating a parvovirus infection, on the other hand, costs over $1,800 dollars or more, and oftentimes the infected pet does not survive. That is why veterinarians promote the use of vaccines in preventative care for pets.

Veterinarians are also very concerned about over-vaccination of pets. That is why most up-to-date veterinarians recommend yearly checking your pet's "titers" to deadly viruses, and only vaccinating when necessary. Alternatives to viral disease prevention such as preparations called "homeopathic nosodes" have been proven to have no effect in preventing infections. Likewise, pet owners can spend around $14 monthly on heartworm prevention, while treatment for the infection often costs $1000 or more. Once dogs are infected with heartworms from mosquitoes, heart failure and kidney failure will result in death.

titers, you can reduce the number of vaccines your dog receives for proper protection. (see some information regarding vaccines in the Resources section). In rare instances pets can have allergic reactions to vaccines. In these situations, these specific vaccines should not be given, and care must be taken to make sure these dogs are protected from any contact with the common deadly viruses, which means only having contact with other dogs that have been vaccinated or keeping your pet in complete isolation indoors.

AVOID ACCESS TO TOXIC BACTERIA IN THE OUTSIDE ENVIRONMENT – USUALLY DECAYING ANIMALS, BIRDS AND REPTILES. **THIS MANY TIMES IS EASIER SAID THAN DONE!**

### Chemical and Environmental Stressors

In today's world, we're literally surrounded by environmental stress in the form of pollution, chemical additives and pesticides. Pollutants are primarily man-made chemicals that don't belong in anyone's body, including your dog's, but have found their way there through contaminated air and water supplies. A growing number of these will pollute the environment and our bodies and our dog's in the future, adding more stress to already overburdened systems.

Dangerous chemicals are everywhere in a dog's environment. And consider this please. Your dog is lower to the ground than you are, placing him

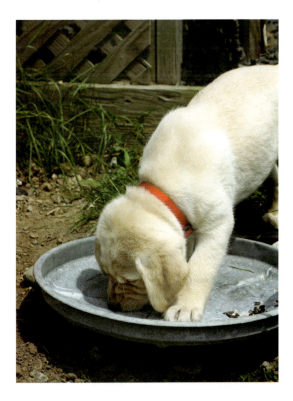

# DR. MURPHY

**Please note**: All medications have positive and negative benefits. When a pet has an acute gastroenteritis from eating a dead toxic squirrel in the back yard - antibiotics, intravenous fluids and other medications are often necessary to save your pet's life! But all of the medications have side effects – like antibiotics upsetting the natural healthy balance of bacterial flora in your dog's colon. Often pets need medications to stay alive, like heart medications when suffering from genetic valvular cardiovascular disease. Even these life-supporting medications can have toxic side effects. We will discuss detox in a future chapter.

or her closer to pesticides in the yard, or along whatever path. This presents your dog many more regular possibilities of encountering pollutants.

Dogs find it great fun to eat almost anything, smell anything and roll in anything – no matter how stinky or rotten in many cases. Bacterial toxins reside in decomposing wildlife that dogs love to eat. Even though bacteria are "natural" some can be deadly. **Additionally, did you realize that new carpet and furniture have been sprayed with fire retardants that are then absorbed into your dog's body?**

Plastic dog chew toys can be "cute" and TOXIC. Your most loving intentions may be riddled with poisons for your dog! Additionally, chemicals are added to many raw hide and other types of treats. Manufacturing practices in many countries are more concerned with producing the lowest cost product and not necessarily a safe product for your pet. Buyer beware has never been more appropriate than with your beloved best friend! Chemicals also find their way into your dog's

body in the form of food additives (approximately 5,000 of them) used to preserve, color, flavor, emulsify and otherwise treat food, both our dog's and our own.

Excessive toxins (chemicals, pollution and drugs) that make their way into the body must be processed and removed. This detoxification process uses large amounts of energy, which leaves little energy for proper digestive function.

Some of these toxins make their way into the bloodstream and continue to circulate there, carrying poisons to the organs. Your dog's resilient liver and kidneys that you learned about in chapter 1 can become overburdened and inefficient at properly detoxifying the body, instigating both acute and chronic disease processes.

## Lowered Production of Enzymes

Ultimately, it comes down to anatomy and physiology. Dog's teeth, as discussed earlier, rip and tear their food with minimal chewing involved. That's why it always seems your dog is gulping down dinner. We humans have special enzymes in our saliva called amylase which begin the job of digestion of carbohydrates (starches) as soon as

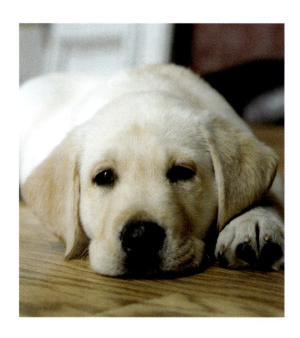

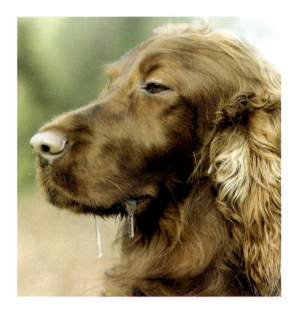

we place food in our mouths. The more efficiently we chew our food, the more complete our carbohydrate digestion can be. Not so with dogs. There is simply no amylase in their saliva. Their saliva is designed to begin the process of killing bacteria and other pathogens they may encounter.

Your dog's food journeys into her stomach where digestion begins. The stomach's job is to initiate the complex project of breaking down proteins (meat). Carbohydrate digestion in a dog (and fat digestion as well) doesn't even happen until the food reaches the small intestine and mixes with pancreatic enzymes. At this point amylase, the carb breakdown enzyme I mentioned earlier, is added into the liquid food contents.

The pancreas produces two types of enzymes – the ones used for digestion of proteins, carbs, and fats and also various others for your dog's metabolic processes (for example, insulin that carries glucose from the bloodstream into the cell).

So what are enzymes anyway? Enzymes are complex proteins that cause chemical changes in other substances. They are the basis of all metabolic activity in the body, facilitating more than 150,000 biochemical reactions and empowering every cell in your dog's body to function.

There are three types of enzymes required by your pet's body: digestive and metabolic enzymes which you've learned come from the pancreas, and food enzymes that must be provided by food sources

- Digestive enzymes - chief of which are protease (digests protein), lipase (for fat digestion) and amylase (for carbohydrate digestion) – break down food into life-giving nutrients.

- Metabolic enzymes take the vitamins, nutrients, and minerals provided by digestive and food enzymes to exactly where they need to go. Every organ requires metabolic enzymes. Your dog's body couldn't function or heal without them. Metabolic enzymes in your dog's bloodstream keep down inflammation.

- Food enzymes also digest food. They are supplied to the body solely through the diet, only from raw foods. Heating food at temperatures of more than 116 degrees destroys food enzymes.

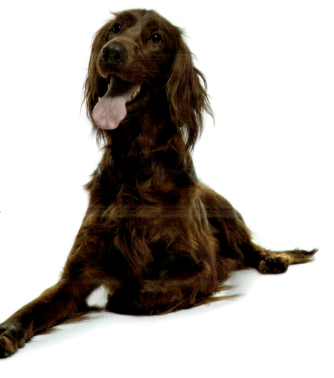

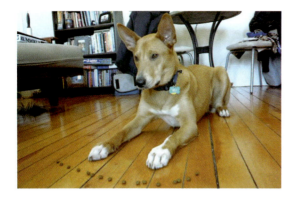

ADDING DIGESTIVE ENZYMES TO YOUR DOG'S MEAL COULD BOOST HIS ABILITY **TO ABSORB VITAL NUTRIENTS LIKE VITAMINS AND MINERALS FROM THEIR FOOD**

Commercial kibble and canned pet foods are processed and heated (as mentioned), therefore, no matter how nutritionally complete the list of foods on the can or package might seem, they are completely devoid of food enzymes. On the other hand, many raw food diets contain only skeletal muscles and bone meal and are also deficient in enzymes.

Let's consider how critical the role of your dog's pancreas is in supporting his healthy digestion.

**As we mentioned in chapter 1, the pancreas:**

- Secretes water and bicarbonates into the duodenum to neutralize the acidity of liquefied food (chyme)
- Secretes enzymes, which break down carbohydrates, protein and fats
- Secretes metabolic enzymes like insulin and glucagon that control sugar metabolism

Enzymes that convert proteins (into amino acids) are the proteases. Part of the job of protease enzymes is to prevent allergic reactions resulting from the absorption through the lining of the gut into the bloodstream of non-digested protein. These non-digested proteins cause an inflammatory immune response in the lymphatic tissue of the intestinal tract. As I've mentioned, healthy lymphatic tissue serves to protect your pet from microbial invaders and toxins. However, inflammation decreases the lymphatic system's protective abilities.

Poor production of the enzymes the pancreas is supposed to produce is a central cause of impaired digestion. Over time, if too much of a drain is put on the pancreas to produce digestive enzymes, production of metabolic enzymes begins to suffer as well. It's the old adage – "stealing from Peter to pay Paul".

Sadly, when enzyme deficiency develops, your pet's immune system is most likely impacted, leading to all sorts of auto-immune diseases not generally seen in generations of dogs in the past. Just as in humans, so many of our diseases like diabetes, heart issues, thyroid and adrenal problems, even cancers have now been linked to poor nutrition.

**Impaired pancreatic function in your dog can result from:**

- Aging
- Physical and mental stress
- Nutritional deficiencies
- A diet of only cooked and processed foods
- Exposure to toxins or radiation
- Genetic weakness and hereditary genetic disease
- Medications
- Infection – bacterial, fungal or parasitic
- Low HCl production in the stomach
- Auto-immune disorders
- Cancer
- Chronic inflammation
- Chronic gastroenteritis
- Small bowel bacterial overgrowth (SIBO)

As we learned in chapter 1, the pancreas also produces insulin and glucagon critical to maintaining a stable blood glucose. Insulin and glucagon are produced after eating, between meals, and during times of illnesses that cause anorexia (loss of appetite).

**Symptoms of pancreatic impairment in your dog could include:**

- Smelly gas
- Indigestion
- Abdominal discomfort
- Bloating
- Food sensitivities
- The presence of undigested fat (and other food) in the stool
- Diarrhea, often with a tan-colored appearance
- Ravenous appetite with weight loss
- In severe pancreatic insufficiency – weight loss, wasting, organ failure and death

## Imbalanced Intestinal  pH

pH is a measurement of acidity/alkalinity. It is measured on a scale from 0 to 14, with substances becoming increasingly more alkaline as the number increases, as per the following table:

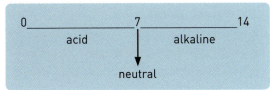

The optimal pH for digestion varies throughout the digestive tract as food moves through it. In the healthy canine digestive tract, the stomach produces extremely acid secretions; the pancreas and gallbladder discharge alkaline juices to buffer the stomach acid; therefore, the small intestine is alkaline, and the colon is normally slightly acidic due to the helpful presence of large populations of bacteria and their fermentation processes.

So, in a healthy system there is a pH shift: acid (stomach) to alkaline (small intestine) to acid (colon). An imbalance of intestinal pH allowing for the growth of bad bacteria, parasites and other microbes can result from:

- Impairment of digestive secretions such as HCl = alkaline (rather than acidic) stomach

- The pancreas failing to produce bicarbonate to alkalize the chyme (partially digested liquidified food) leaving the stomach and entering the duodenum = acidic (rather than alkaline) small intestine.

- Antacids given habitually in attempts to decrease heartburn (even dogs are given antacids for symptoms of heartburn) = alkaline (rather than acidic) stomach

If the pH of any of the key digestive organs is out of balance, the result will be impaired digestion and its adverse health consequences, beginning with bacterial imbalance, unbalanced intestinal environment overall, and leading to any number of chronic degenerative diseases in your dog.

I hope you're beginning to understand that impaired digestion can begin in many ways, any of which can set your dog on the path to declining health over time.

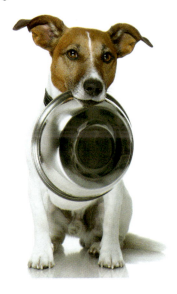

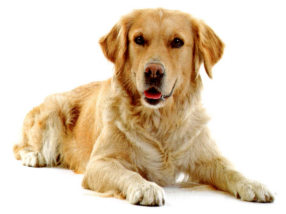

## PROCESS OF DECLINING HEALTH

**Impaired Digestion**

**Imbalance of Gut Flora**

**Intestinal Toxemia**

**Leaky Gut**

**Chronic Disease**

Probiotics are the "good" bacteria that populate the small and large intestines of all humans and also our dogs. The word "probiotic" means "for life". These beneficial bacteria play a key role in your dog's health. Because nearly 75% of your dog's immune defenses are located in the digestive tract, having the proper balance of intestinal bacteria is an essential part of achieving and maintaining overall health.

When your dog does not have enough probiotics in their digestive tract the bad (pathogenic) bacteria can take over the gut environment. This can eventually lead to an imbalance of gut flora and a decline in both gut and overall wellness. As I've mentioned before, your dog's digestive tract is the core of his overall health.

## IMBALANCE OF GUT FLORA

The next step in our flow chart of declining health involves the imbalance of gut flora, the inevitable result of impaired digestion.

The microflora composition of the intestinal tract is complex. There is a simple way to understand the different bacteria groupings in the gut: In every dog there is a ratio of good (health-promoting) bacteria, neutral bacteria (commensal) and pathogenic (disease-causing) bacteria. All of these organisms are competing for food and space in the digestive tract.

It is important that the good bacteria be abundant in the digestive tract. When the microbial population becomes unbalanced, disease-causing bacteria may dominate. For example, if fungal overgrowth (which is a natural inhabitant of the gut) or some other microbe grows out of control, the gut flora is out of balance.

**Here are a few of the ways that good bacteria (probiotics) benefit your dog's health:**

- They assist in the digestion and absorption of essential nutrients
- Probiotics support the immune system
- Good bacteria promote intestinal well-being
- They help maintain healthy bowel function
- They nourish and balance the other natural gut bacteria
- They assist in the process of regularly restoring and rebuilding the digestive tract

Fortunately, there are many ways to correct and maintain the critical balance of good to bad bacteria in your dog's digestive system. Keep reading. We will discuss this in detail in an upcoming chapter.

**The primary factors that cause imbalanced gut flora are:**

- **Antibiotics** – This term literally means "anti-life". Antibiotics do not discriminate They kill the disease-causing bacteria as well as the good bacteria in the gut, disrupting the bacterial balance overall. Even many vets still do not fully understand the importance of maintaining bacterial balance in your dog's digestive tract. It is important that you make sure it is absolutely necessary for your pet to take an antibiotic should one be suggested.

- **Medications** like steroids – prednisone, cortisone, and others

- **Poor diet** – As we've discussed, many dog foods on the store shelves are deficient in the nutrients your dog requires to maintain health. Remember that probiotics are destroyed in any type of heating process, so even if a food or treat claims to contain probiotics, the chances are slim that any live through the packaging process.

- **Stress** – In dogs just like with humans, stress and anxiety can disrupt the good to bad bacteria balance in the gut.

- **Vaccinations** – Although necessary, vaccinations can affect the dog's immune system and lower the good bacteria levels. These days, it is becoming more common for vets to test a vaccine titer in your dog, establishing whether an additional vaccine is really needed at that time.

**The critical balance of good to bad bacteria can be maintained if:**

- The immune system is functioning normally.

- An optimal ratio of "good"/neutral to "bad" bacteria (80:20) is maintained.

- The pH of the colon is balanced (on the slightly acid side).

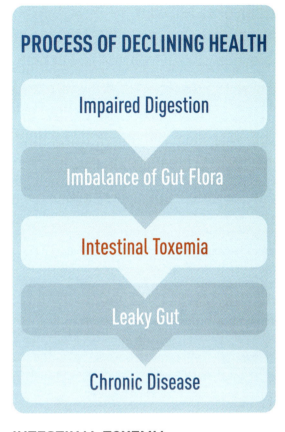

## PROCESS OF DECLINING HEALTH

Impaired Digestion

Imbalance of Gut Flora

Intestinal Toxemia

Leaky Gut

Chronic Disease

## INTESTINAL TOXEMIA

To this point we've seen how impaired digestion over time leads to an imbalance of intestinal flora. Once your dog's "good" to "bad" bacteria are out of balance, this paves the way for intestinal toxemia – poisoning of the intestines.

We typically think we swallow food and it just breaks down into nutrients like magic! When you follow the food down the digestive tube as we have been doing, you see there are many enzymatic chemical processes that must occur to turn the food into something that can actually feed and maintain your dog's cells and tissues.

Intestinal toxemia initially is the chemical result of bad bacteria acting on undigested food. This interaction produces toxic chemicals and gases. Essentially, food becomes a toxin itself!

These nasty chemicals and gases are called endotoxins - poisons from within. They are

**THINK OF IT THIS WAY.** THE BUILDUP OF TOXINS CHANGES THE GUT NEIGHBORHOOD INTERNALLY. YOU DOG'S GUT NEIGHBORHOOD TRANSITIONS FROM NICE SINGLE-FAMILY HOMES WITH PLEASANT SCHOOLS AND GROCERY STORES TO ONE THAT IS FILLED WITH BARS AND UNSAVORY CHARACTERS. LOTS OF FERMENTATION HAPPENS (THINK BEER AND SMOKE?). **I KNOW BY NOW YOU'RE LAUGHING, BUT HOPEFULLY THIS WILL HELP YOU UNDERSTAND HOW IMPORTANT MAINTAINING YOUR PET'S INTERNAL NEIGHBORHOOD CAN BE.**

produced as a byproduct of impaired digestion and imbalance of gut flora. Endotoxins are just as damaging to the body as the external environmental toxins like pesticides and other chemicals called exotoxins that we've discussed previously.

These toxins can damage the delicate mucosal lining, resulting in increased intestinal permeability (leaky gut), which we will explore further as the next step in declining health. The net result is that the toxins are then able to gain access to the bloodstream, spreading throughout the body and creating inflammation in their wake.

Endotoxins can also produce free radicals which cause serious damage to cells when they rip electrons out of cell membranes. Free radicals live only momentarily, but can do a great amount of damage in that short period of time. Large numbers of free radicals are produced by dozens of intestinal toxins.

TO DEACTIVATE FREE RADICALS, THE BODY DEPLOYS ANTIOXIDANTS, NUTRIENTS THAT ACT AS FREE RADICAL SCAVENGERS. **VITAMINS A, C AND E AND THE MINERALS SELENIUM AND ZINC ARE WELL KNOWN ANTIOXIDANTS.** THIS IS WHY SUPPLEMENTING WITH A MULTIVITAMIN IS OFTEN A GOOD CHOICE FOR YOUR DOG ON A DAILY BASIS.

What is not so well known is that the bile produced by the liver has very powerful free radical scavenging effects. The healthy liver and gallbladder function which we explored in chapter 1 is critical in preventing free radical damage. We'll discuss how to protect these vital organs in a future chapter.

**Bottom line** - the situation looks like this - In the beginning stages of intestinal toxemia, your dog's body generally has sufficient nutritional reserves to manage the various stressors. At this point, he is not acutely distressed, and symptoms may not be apparent.

## DR. MURPHY

Even low-grade bacterial toxemia causes severe inflammation in the intestinal tract but also on your pet's body in other ways.

- Chronic inflammation in the liver – called chronic active hepatitis

- Damage to the kidneys – the kidneys cannot regenerate and chronic exposure to bacterial toxins causes progressive damage to the kidney. Kidney failure is one of the leading causes of death in dogs.

- Chronic over-stimulation to the intestinal immune system (80% of the dog's immune system) that can result in overall immune system malfunction and diseases such as: autoimmune disease, allergies, damage to joints from arthritis, premature aging, cancer.

**ENDOTOXINS WHICH ARE INTERNALLY PRODUCED ARE CARRIED TO THE LIVER BY THE BLOODSTREAM.** THEY PROCEED FROM THERE TO OTHER ORGANS OF THE BODY—THE BRAIN, NERVOUS SYSTEM, JOINTS, SKIN, ETC. IF THE LIVER'S DETOXIFICATION ABILITY IS IMPAIRED DUE TO INADEQUATE NUTRITION AND TOXIC OVERLOAD, THESE TOXINS WILL BE STORED AND OFTEN INITIATE CHRONIC ILLNESS.

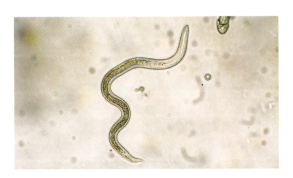

### Parasites

Because of dog behavior and frequent exposure, parasites have always been one of the major maladies of dogs. Until very recent times parasites and viruses were the most common cause of death in dogs. Veterinary medical advances with vaccines and safe parasite treatments have had the biggest impact on the health and longevity of our pets. Parasite infections are one of the most common problems veterinarians find on their examination of dogs.

As we take a look at both how and why our pets may contract parasites, please realize that many of the dog parasitic infections can be transmitted to people and cause very serious health conditions.

Intestinal parasites such as hookworms, round worms, coccidia, and giardia cause severe damage to the intestinal tract as well as other organs and cause symptoms such as weight loss, vomiting, diarrhea, poor hair coat and generalized debilitation in our pets. This is why veterinarians check puppies for parasites at every visit and check adult dogs at least once a year.

Parasitic infestations are very common and when diagnosed early are easily treated. Left untreated however, parasites will continue to multiply and produce both damage to the intestinal tract as well as digestive functions. The resulting inflammation and physical damage to the intestinal mucosa leads to intestinal toxemia, unhealthy bacterial overgrowth and even more serious inflammation.

IN MANY CASES, YOUR DOG'S ABILITY TO COMBAT VARIOUS PARASITES IS **IS BASED UPON THE HEALTH OF THE GUT AND THE STRENGTH OF YOUR DOG'S IMMUNE SYSTEM.**

In a nutshell, all these various interactions result in intestinal toxemia, inflammation of the intestinal wall and the breakdown in function of the intestinal lining (mucosa), with the eventual appearance of various chronic and seemingly "age-related" disorders which we'll discuss in our next chapter.

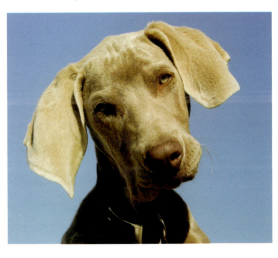

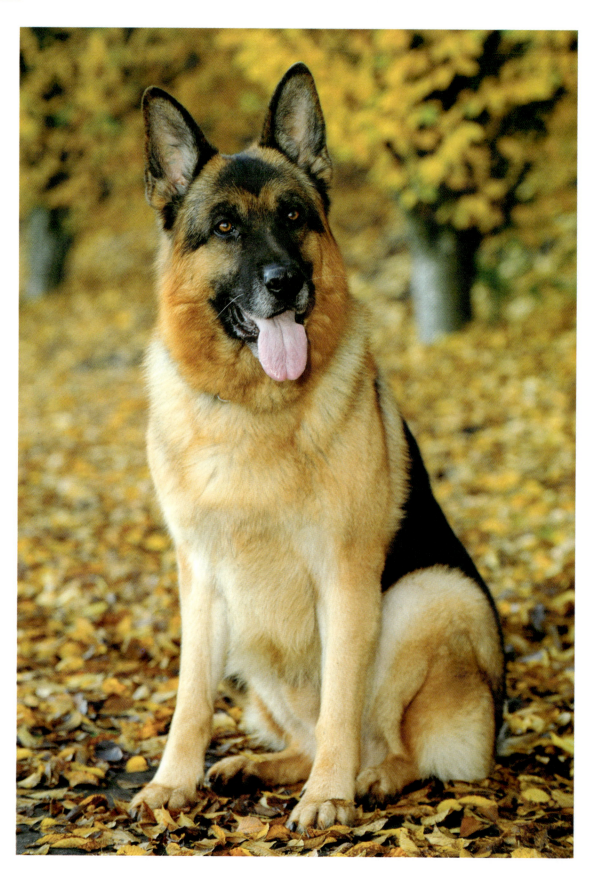

## CHAPTER 3

# LEAKY GUT SYNDROM AND CHRONIC DISEASE

Leaky Gut Syndrome (also known as intestinal permeability) describes the inevitable result of impaired digestion, imbalanced gut flora and intestinal toxemia.

What exactly is a leaky gut anyway? As you know, the healthy mucous lining of the small intestine is a semi-permeable membrane that allows nutrients like vitamins, minerals and antioxidants to enter the bloodstream, while shielding it from unwanted toxins like parasites, other pathogenic organisms and undigested food proteins. This mucous lining is like the screen on a window in a house that lets the air in but keeps the bugs out. It is also like the skin, in that it sloughs off a layer of cells naturally every three to five days and produces new cells to keep the lining semi-permeable.

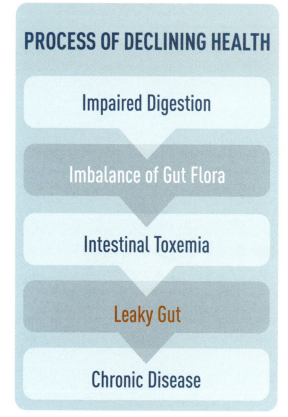

## PROCESS OF DECLINING HEALTH

Impaired Digestion

Imbalance of Gut Flora

Intestinal Toxemia

Leaky Gut

Chronic Disease

Once the steps to declining health we've discussed have eroded this membrane, it becomes permeable. (The "screen" on the "window" becomes filled with holes, letting the pests into the patio!) You can imagine that the lining itself under these toxic conditions is quite inflamed.

The damaged intestinal lining allows unwanted toxins, proteins and big food particles to pass between your dog's intestine and his bloodstream. These substances actually don't belong in the bloodstream, although they might be substances that aren't immediately harmful.

The primary role of the immune system is to defend the body against foreign invaders or abnormal cells that invade or attack it.

Soon the immune system attacks these inappropriate substances, tagging them as foreign invaders and develops antibodies (chemical bullets) against them. Powerful inflammatory chemicals are released by the immune system such as histamine, leukotrines, cytokines and prostaglandins.

The immune system of the intestinal tract is the largest part of your dog's immune system and has to deal with all of these proteins and chemicals that have crossed over the mucous membranes into the bloodstream. This results in a chronically over stimulated immune system that starts becoming over reactive to everything in the environment such as pollens and molds in the air.

The chemical responses of the over stimulated immune system result in either overt allergic responses (like itching and dermatitis, runny eyes, ear infections) or silent inflammatory issues internally resulting in auto-immune conditions. Simply stated, your dog's body is attacking itself!

Additionally, when the intestinal lining can no longer absorb key nutrients efficiently, nutritional deficiencies can unfortunately result in chronic disease processes.

The following symptoms may or may not be recognized as the result of leaky gut syndrome, since symptoms can occur anywhere in the body. Our dogs can't voice their symptoms, which makes it even more difficult for us to know what's going on inside. This unseen and unheard vicious cycle can continue for months and years.

- Gas
- Cramps
- Bloating
- Constipation
- Vomiting
- Diarrhea
- Skin disorders
- Various inflammatory bowel diseases (IBD)
- Joint and muscle pain
- Bad breath

# DIGESTIVE CARE

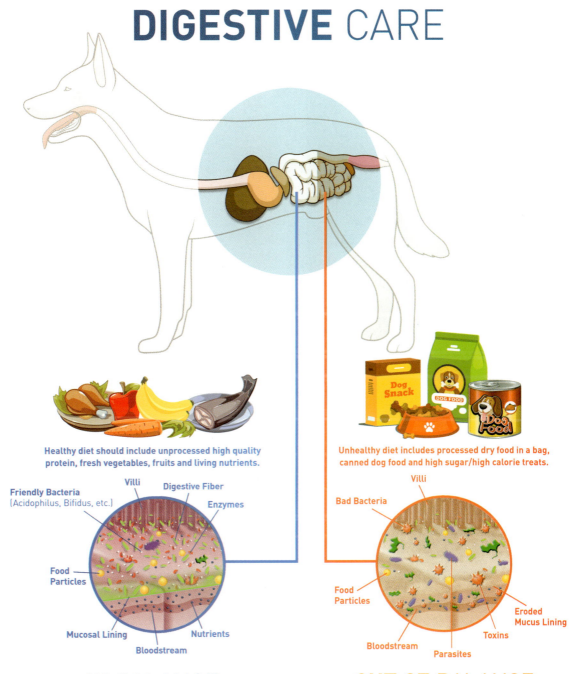

Healthy diet should include unprocessed high quality protein, fresh vegetables, fruits and living nutrients.

Unhealthy diet includes processed dry food in a bag, canned dog food and high sugar/high calorie treats.

**Friendly Bacteria** (Acidophilus, Bifidus, etc.)

**Villi**

**Digestive Fiber**

**Enzymes**

**Food Particles**

**Mucosal Lining**

**Nutrients**

**Bloodstream**

**Bad Bacteria**

**Villi**

**Food Particles**

**Bloodstream**

**Parasites**

**Toxins**

**Eroded Mucus Lining**

## IN BALANCE

A healthy digestive tract has a semi-permeable mucosal lining that helps prevent undigested food and toxins from entering the bloodstream. Fully digested nutrients and liquids may pass through to nourish the body.

## OUT OF BALANCE

An out-of-balance digestive tract can have a porous mucosal lining. Undigested foods and toxins can pass through to enter the bloodstream.

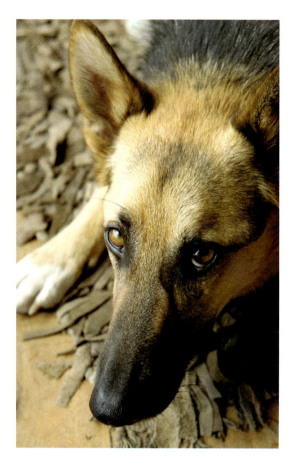

Leaky gut can also be aggravated by a number of other factors that I've mentioned previously that can cause the earlier stages of distressed digestive health. Are you beginning to notice a similarity in causes of all levels of declining overall health?

**Factors contributing to Leaky Gut**

- Foods too high in carbohydrates and/or fats
- Parasites
- Bacterial infections
- Bacterial Toxins – spoiled food
- Viral Diseases
- Eating indigestible material
- Toxic plants
- Chemicals (in processed foods)
- Environmental chemicals (like pesticides)
- Enzyme deficiencies
- Corticosteroids
- Antibiotics
- NSAIDs (Non-Steroidal Anti-Inflammatory Drugs)

Declining digestive health in humans manifests in conditions like fatigue, headaches, memory loss, poor concentration and irritability. It makes sense that a dog could experience the same, and be unable to express the discomfort in a way a pet parent might understand.

**Although the veterinary community doesn't often address leaky gut syndrome as a primary issue, the breakdown of the intestinal lining is absolutely a precursor of chronic inflammatory conditions and age-related diseases. Understanding will help you to recognize and overcome early warning signs in your dog.**

**Leaky gut syndrome can manifest in malabsorption of many important nutrients:**

- Vitamins
- Minerals
- Amino acids

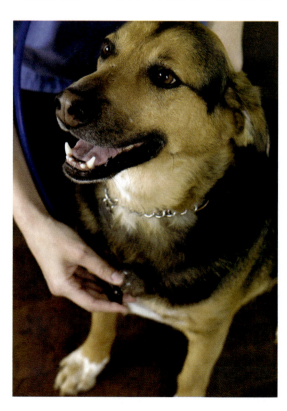

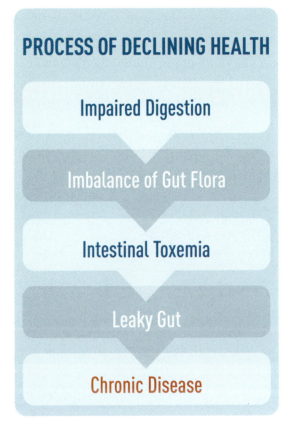

# PROCESS OF DECLINING HEALTH

**Impaired Digestion**

**Imbalance of Gut Flora**

**Intestinal Toxemia**

**Leaky Gut**

**Chronic Disease**

## CHRONIC DISEASE

Ultimately, your dog begins to show symptoms of chronic conditions specific to her situation and genetic predisposition like:

**Allergies and Food Sensitivities**
• Skin and coat issues
**Inflammatory Intestinal Disorders**
• SIBO
• IBS
• Colitis (IBD)
**Kidney, Pancreas and/or Liver Issues**
**Arthritis and Joint Disorders**

Sadly, many times you'll be told that the cause of many chronic conditions is "unknown" by many traditional veterinary and medical doctors. However, I'm here to tell you that things are changing!

Alternative physicians are becoming increasingly aware of the importance of the GI tract in the development of chronic disease and allergy. In fact, researchers now estimate that half to two thirds of all immune activity occurs in the gut.

## Allergies and Food Sensitivities

For both humans and dogs, the words "allergy" or "sensitivity" can bring up confusion on many levels. For the sake of our conversation I am going to use the two terms somewhat interchangeably, as that is most likely how you will see them when reading further on this subject.

Most important to determine is the cause of your dog's unhappy symptoms environmental? For example, pollen or something else contacted in the indoors or out? Or do the irritating symptoms relate to something that has been eaten – perhaps a food or a treat? Even a dog bowl, toys or bedding can cause issues for some dogs, so let's try to understand a bit more about the process leading to allergies/sensitivities.

Technically, it is very rare for a dog to have a true food allergy which manifests as an itchy dermatitis. In humans this is recognized in the extreme by the possibility of anaphylactic shock, example: when an allergic person eats peanuts. Instead, dogs will more commonly become allergic to pollens and molds – manifesting in itchy inflamed skin with secondary bacterial and fungal skin diseases.

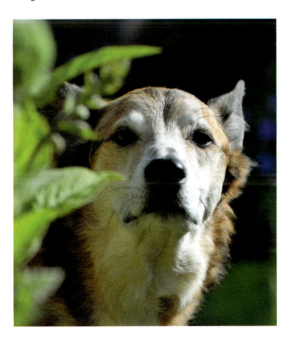

An immune attack begins with the body producing antibodies (chemical bullets), which bind to the foreign invaders, forming what are known as immune complexes. These cause the body's reactions that result in an experience of the diverse and unpleasant symptoms we recognize as allergies or food sensitivities.

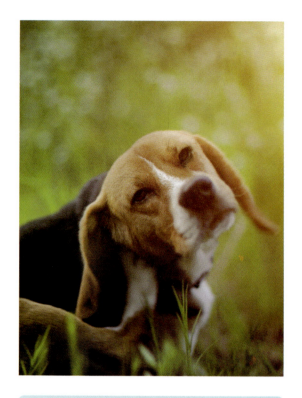

**Symptoms of allergy or food sensitivity you may notice in your dog:**

- Itchy ears and ear infections
- Increased scratching of skin
- Chewing on paws/swollen paws
- Red, moist or scabbed skin from scratching
- Persistent licking
- Irritated, runny eyes
- Itchy back or base of tail (commonly a flea allergy)
- Sneezing
- Increased snoring due to an inflamed throat
- Vomiting
- Diarrhea
- Secondary bacterial or yeast skin infections, which may cause hair loss, scabs or crusts on the skin.

IMPORTANT NOTE! SENSITIVITIES AND ALLERGIES MAY DEVELOP IN RESPONSE TO ANYTHING IN THE ENVIRONMENT—INCLUDING FOOD. THE RESPONSE TO THE IRRITANT— BE IT CORN OR PETROCHEMICALS, NEW CARPET OR A DOG TOY, EVEN FOOD ADDITIVES—CAN AFFECT ANY ORGAN OF THE BODY. THE GUT WILL ALWAYS BE INVOLVED, HOWEVER.

**What causes the immune system to become unbalanced and over-responsive?**

- Toxins – ex: exposure to chemicals, plastics
- Bacteria and bacterial toxins
- Viral diseases
- Parasitic infection
- Malnutrition or poor nutrition
- Vitamin deficiencies like vitamins A, E, D, selenium
- Unbalanced gut bacteria (microbiota)
- Hormonal deficiency or imbalance – such as hypothyroid
- Hyperadrenocorticism – Cushing's disease
- Diabetes mellitus
- Processed foods
- Genetic disorders
- Emotional imbalance: chronic stress, fear, anxiety
- Many drugs
- Over-vaccination
- Cancer

IN HUMANS, ALLERGY SYMPTOMS ARE OFTEN ASSOCIATED WITH SNEEZING, ITCHY MEMBRANES, PERHAPS RED EYES, SKIN IRRITATION. HOWEVER, **IF YOUR DOG HAS DEVELOPED AN "ALLERGY", MOST LIKELY HE WILL BE PLAGUED BY ITCHY OR INFLAMED SKIN, USUALLY WITH SECONDARY SKIN AND EAR BACTERIAL AND FUNGAL INFECTIONS.**

## DR. MURPHY

Of all of the skin and coat issues that may affect dogs, allergic dermatitis is the most common. Allergic dermatitis causes immense suffering in dogs, prompting them to itch and scratch excessively. The more dogs itch and scratch themselves, the worse the dermatitis. This creates a cycle of pain and trauma. Secondary to the inflammation in the skin and self-induced trauma, surface bacteria invade the skin, in turn causing more itching, scratching and self-induced trauma.

**Allergic dermatitis can be the result of inappropriate reaction to:**

- Fleas
- Atopy (caused by inhaling pollen, mold, etc.)
- Contact allergies
- Food allergies
- Unusual reaction to medications
- Secondary yeast infections

In humans, we use the catch-all phrase "candida" which is an overgrowth of a specific yeast in the digestive system in humans. While gut candida infection are very rare in dogs, other yeast infections are very widespread. The primary yeast infection in dogs is Malassezia.

When dogs have allergies commonly the external ear is almost always affected. The inflammation in the ear from allergy creates a perfect condition for bacteria and Malassezia to grow. The Malassezia creates even more inflammation resulting in a chronic progressive otitis (inflammation of the ear).

Allergic otitis with secondary Malassezia and bacterial infections is one of the most common dog maladies treated by veterinarians. If detected early and treated effectively – which includes maintenance treatment for the underlying allergy, atopic allergic otitis is easily treated and the ear returns to normal. Left untreated severe inflammation and changes in the cartilage and can be a very painful disease that is difficult and expensive to manage. In very severe cases, surgery may be necessary to remove the entire ear, solving the infection and pain but resulting in deafness.

Itchy skin diseases such as allergies to pollens and molds cause inflammation. Yeast infections invade the dogs skin, especially when the skin is compromised by allergies and other dermatitis. It is important to treat both the allergy and the yeast infection to make your dog comfortable again.

**IF YOU NOTICE THAT YOUR DOG IS ITCHY IN THE SPRING AND FALL, OR HE ONLY SCRATCHES WHEN HE'S IN CERTAIN PLACES,** IT'S LIKELY HE MAY BE ALLERGIC TO POLLEN OR DUST.

Food allergies appear when the body develops antibodies to the (undigested) proteins derived from previously harmless food (remember how the food gets through the bug screen?).

Proteins are found in almost all foods. In fact, non-sprouted grains proteins are one of the worst enemies of your dog's intestinal lining!

**TIP**     **Wheat and other grains contain protein!**

The dog's leaky gut allows the irritants to enter any tissue and trigger an inflammatory reaction when that food is eaten.

**YOUR DOG CAN BECOME SENSITIVE TO ANY FOOD – EVEN FOODS THAT YOU BELIEVE ARE EXTREMELY HEALTHY AND SUPPORTIVE (AND EXPENSIVE).**

## Inflammatory Intestinal Disorders

Sadly, as the name implies, these conditions are obviously gut-related and much more common in dogs than you or I would care to believe.

Inflammatory intestinal disorders are simply the next step in the Process of Declining Health. The inflammation has advanced to a more serious and exhausting level of illness. With a disorder of this nature, it's critical to determine the specific issue through veterinary testing at this

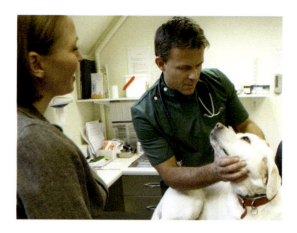

point in order to determine appropriate treatment protocols. These intestinal conditions, once they reach this point of suffering, are now given specific names beyond the term "digestive issues".

**Here is a list of symptoms that your dog may experience with these types of disorders:**

- Diarrhea
- Fatigue
- Weight loss
- Rumbling and gurgling abdominal sounds from the abdomen
- Loss of interest in daily activities
- Chronic recurrent vomiting
- Chronic or smelly gas
- Abdominal tenderness
- Constipation
- Bright red blood in stool
- Distressed coat hair

**Let's take a quick look at a few of these named conditions.**

**Small Intestinal Bacterial Overgrowth** (SIBO)

Although the majority of bacteria are found in the large intestine (colon), a small amount of bacteria in the small intestine is critical for the production and absorption of certain B vitamins. When these bacteria multiply profusely due to various issues, many of which we've already explored, your dog can manifest SIBO, which

## BRENDA WATSON

While studying the effects of probiotics on dogs, I was fortunate to interview Dr. Jan S. Suchodolski and his assistant at the Texas A&M Small Animal Hospital. They were actively conducting research on the efficacy of probiotics used to resolve gastrointestinal issues like IBD (Inflammatory Bowel Disease).

In this veterinary hospital, no matter what the dog's symptoms might be, blood tests are performed evaluating bowel function.

The day I was there, I had the opportunity to sit in on a follow-up office visit with a woman who had brought her Sheltie in with an eye problem. Bloodwork was performed initially and much to the surprise of the pet parent, her dog was diagnosed with IBD! Her dog had not exhibited any GI symptoms whatsoever!

The treatment prescribed for the Sheltie was dietary change and oral probiotics. It was so interesting to hear that her dog was now free of any eye issues, and her follow-up bloodwork showed that the IBD was on the mend.

In my experience, this scenario happens frequently in humans. Over the years, people have asked me about issues with their skin, ears, eyes, joints and nervous systems. When I questioned them about experiencing any digestive issues like gas, bloating, constipation, diarrhea – they have answered me that they had absolutely no symptoms. Like the veterinarians at Texas A&M, I suggested dietary change and probiotics and I'm so happy to tell you that their issues began to resolve as well.

dramatically impacts digestive function. One clue that your dog might be experiencing this condition is smelly bad breath (not due to dental issues).

**Irritable Bowel Syndrome** (IBS)

IBS refers to a chronic condition in dogs with diarrhea, constipation, pain, bloating, lethargy and loss of appetite. Usually no pathological lesions can be found on diagnostic tests. This condition is most often considered to be stress or diet related, and interestingly a lack of dietary fiber which can stabilize the intestinal microbiota is causative in some cases.

**Inflammatory Bowel Disease** (IBD)

Chronic inflammation of the small intestine resulting in thickened intestinal mucosa in the small intestine and abnormal digestion.

The result is extreme food (protein) sensitivity with frequent vomiting and diarrhea. **Chronic inflammation causes the GI immune system, then the entire immune system to become over-stimulated. An overstimulated immune system results in a cascade of unhealthy processes in your pet.**

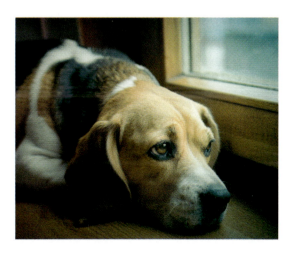

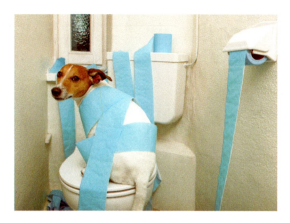

**Chronic Colitis**

Colitis is one of the most serious digestive diseases and can be life-threatening. This debilitating disease can have many unresolved underlying causes as previously discussed. Chronic colitis results in chronic diarrhea, bloody diarrhea, accidents in the house, discomfort and pain.

Chronic inflammation of the colon results in the GI immune system in a constant state of over stimulation. This can be the underlying cause of skin allergies and worse life threatening autoimmune disorders.

The colon is also the home to trillions of bacteria. When the colon is inflamed and the colon mucosa is disrupted these bacteria can invade the body resulting in blood poisoning (septicemia).

With any intestinal inflammatory condition, nutritional deficiencies are very common, due to the irritated condition of the small intestine resulting in your dog's reduced ability to absorb vital nutrition.

To list all the conditions that can initiate a disruption in normal digestive habits is beyond the scope of this book. My intention here is to help you understand how similar the causes of declining health are. The symptoms that manifest are very similar as well. That's why it's so important to observe your dog's

behaviors and bowel habits and contact your vet should your pet experience any shift in either for any length of time. Intestinal damage along with abatement of symptoms can happen quickly with an appropriate treatment protocol, however it's imperative to determine the root cause of the changes. Please don't allow digestive disorders to become chronic and debilitating for your dear pet.

## Kidney, Pancreas and/or Liver Issues

### Kidney

In dogs the organ that often fails the first is the kidneys. Constant inflammation from bacterial overgrowth and bacterial toxins from your pet's mouth is a common cause of kidney failure in dogs. Trillions of unhealthy bacteria attack the mucosa every day invading the rich blood supply of the mouth. In dogs the kidneys bear the brunt of these toxins. Bacterial dental disease is preventable with routine dental care. This is why routine dental care for your dog is such a priority for veterinarians.

# DR. MURPHY

Another cause of chronic kidney failure is chronic systemic inflammation as caused by chronic intestinal disease. Chronic systemic inflammation from intestinal disease can cause, exacerbate and accelerate chronic renal failure - the most common kidney disease in dogs. In this disease the functional kidney filtering system is replaced with scar tissue. As the kidney fails, toxins normally excreted by the kidneys build up in the body. The most sensitive tissue in the body to these toxins is the intestinal mucosa. This results in loss of appetite, vomiting and diarrhea, weight loss and rapid degeneration of intestinal mucosal health.

GOOD DENTAL CARE, PREVENTING AND TREATING INFECTED GUMS AND TEETH **IS KEY IN PROTECTING YOUR DOG AGAINST CHRONIC KIDNEY ISSUES.**

### Pancreas

The pancreas is a vital and interconnected organ of the intestinal tract. Bacterial toxins, SIBO, and intestinal disease often affects and involves the pancreas.

The pancreas produces and stores powerful enzymes. These enzymes are inactivated in the pancreas and activated when released into the small intestines. The process is similar to mixing the different parts of epoxy glue together for activation.

In some cases, chronic low-grade inflammation or immune system imbalance causes the pancreas to stop functioning. Pancreatic insufficiency causes even more intestinal mucosal disease, malabsorption disease, and eventually malnutrition and death.

## DR. MURPHY

When the pancreas is inflamed, inappropriate pancreatic enzymes are released and activated in the intestines. This causes severe inflammation resulting in the release of even more enzymes and serious life-threatening inflammation. Without aggressive intravenous therapy, dogs often die.

### Liver

The liver is the central organ of detoxification of toxins both in the body and from the intestinal tract. The liver is also responsible for taking all the nutrients absorbed by the intestinal tract

as raw ingredients and making the proteins essential for body tissue repair and health. The liver plays a huge role in your pet's immune system.

An unhealthy intestinal tract results in an unhealthy liver and vice versa. When the liver is lacking in vital health every cell in the body is affected adversely.

## DR. MURPHY

Veterinarians often suspect liver dysfunction in dogs that have frequent vomiting and diarrhea. Dogs with liver failure or sub-optimal liver function (as in portal caval shunts) often have an allergic reaction to vaccines.

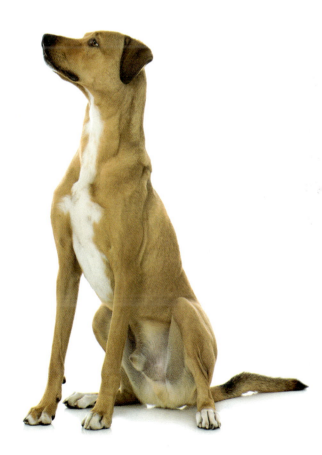

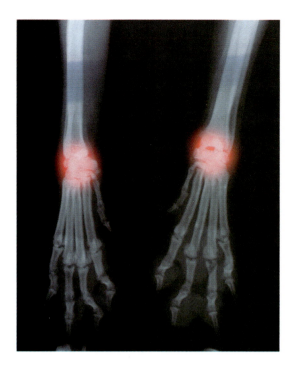

## Arthritis and Joint Disorders

Arthritis is probably one of the most common seemingly age-related chronic conditions experienced by both humans and their beloved four-legged friends. I say "seemingly age-related" because the inflammatory changes that define this degenerative condition can actually begin at a very young age. Happily, many cases of this debilitating condition can be prevented, or if already present, can be supported to heal in a very positive direction which I will share with you.

The word "arthritis" breaks into "arth" meaning "joint" and "itis" which means inflammation or irritation. So you see, arthritis is simply inflammation or irritation of a joint space, differing from an inevitable scary disease. However, that inflammation can result in a lot of pain and decreased mobility for your pet.

Do you remember how the toxic substances can travel into the bloodstream through a leaky gut, and then travel throughout the body? One of the most common places those inflammatory compounds deposit is in the joints. Over time these toxins can result in osteoarthritis.

This is not to say that all arthritis is caused by chronic inflammation. There are different types and causes of arthritis. Some breeds have genetic tendencies toward joint problems and they may experience symptoms at an early age. We've all felt heartbroken when we see German Shepherd and Labradors with genetic debilitating hip issues. Some arthritis is the result of injuries.

To complicate the situation even further, the medications that are commonly prescribed to relieve painful arthritic and joint conditions are the same drugs that can cause leaky gut, which as you now understand, leads to even more inflammation and a progression of the degenerative process.

Personally, I wonder if this particular degenerative condition might be stayed for many years if the pet parents had been aware of the importance of digestive health when they brought their puppy home and implemented the preventative measures I'm excited to share with you in future chapters of this book.

## DR. MURPHY

It can be a catch-22. To reduce inflammation in the joints veterinarians used to use corticosteroids but these drugs can have many side effects. NSAIDS used by humans such as aspirin, tylenol and ibuprofen are very toxic to dogs and even small doses cause serious injury to the intestinal mucosa. Safer NSAIDS such as carprofen and metacam are used by veterinarians but still have clinical and subclinical effects on the intestinal mucosa. Newer medications for arthritis such as grapiprant have minimal effects to no adverse effects on the intestinal mucosa.

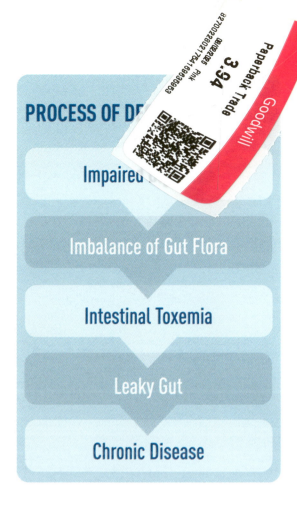

## PROCESS OF DE...

Impaired...

Imbalance of Gut Flora

Intestinal Toxemia

Leaky Gut

Chronic Disease

## A Quick Recap

As our Process of Declining Health flow chart indicates, impaired digestion leads to imbalanced gut flora, wherein bacteria act upon undigested food in the gut, producing endotoxins. Intestinal toxemia can lead to an overgrowth of bad bacteria, viruses and various parasites. Proliferation of these opportunistic organisms creates more unbalanced gut flora in the intestines causing irritation of the intestinal tract, tissue damage and impaired circulation, any of which can lead to gastrointestinal inflammation.

Leaky gut syndrome occurs when the intestinal lining becomes porous and irritated. As time passes, the breakdown in the lining can result in the passage of undigested food particles, toxins and parasites into the bloodstream leading to a weakened immune system, allergies, digestive disorders and, eventually, chronic disease.

Please do not be dismayed by our study of the Process of Declining Health! You, an informed pet parent, are your dog's best insurance for a long and happy life.

You'll be excited to hear that the rest of this book is dedicated to showing you the way to make sure your dog has the healthiest and most vital digestive and immune systems possible – starting from wherever he or she may be on his or her health journey today.

Bottom line, whether the breed of dog you love is genetically inclined toward arthritic conditions, or if your pet is young or old, there will never be a more important time than now for you to understand how gut health is connected to overall health and make a decision to provide your best friend with the best preventative or supportive care measures that are available on this planet – soon to come!

As you can see, even with these few examples of chronic diseases that I've mentioned, digestive and behavioral issues can forecast serious conditions for your dog in the future, or in some cases, immediately. Always keep your vet's phone number close. If you're anything like me, your dog is your furry child, and you would always choose for him or her to be feeling great at all times. After all, when they feel wonderful, their enthusiasm and love rubs off on you too!

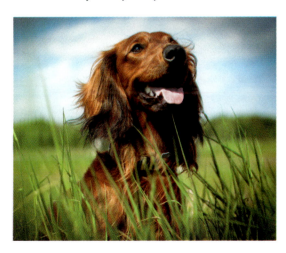

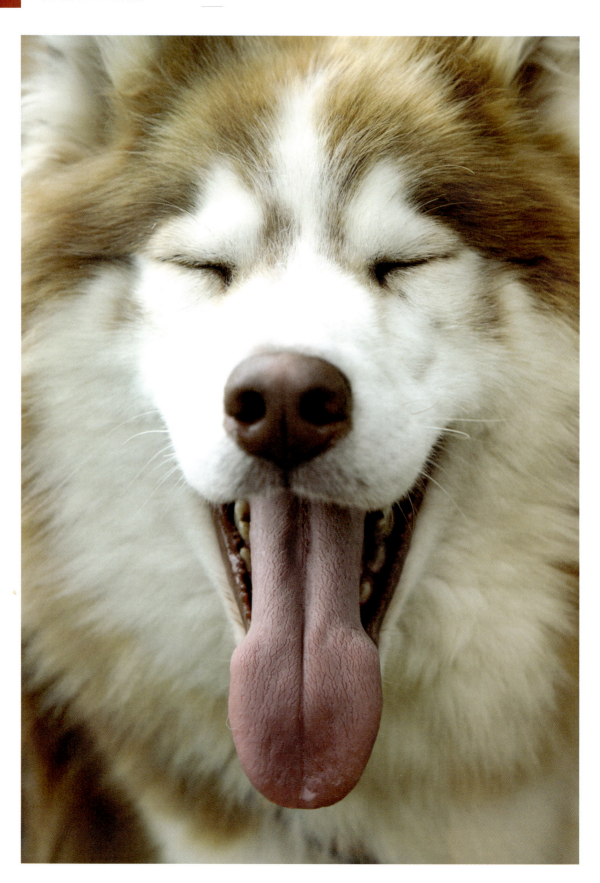

## CHAPTER 4

# H.O.P.E. AND **MORE**
# FOR THE FUTURE

I'm excited to share guidelines that enhance the digestive process in the rest of this book, which you now understand is the first step in the prevention of disease as your dog ages. The process of healing and restoring the body to health involves taking certain steps and maintaining good health requires wise choices. Health is not just the absence of symptoms or pain for your pet. Health is defined in terms of the whole dog, not in terms of diseased body parts.

# VITAL SOLUTIONS
## FOR YOUR DOG

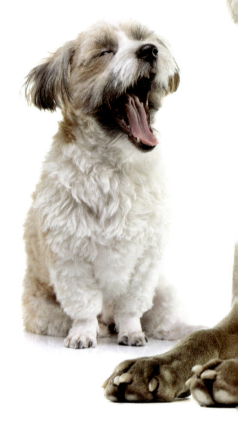

**VITAL HEALTH**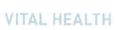

High Energy

Ideal Weight

Detoxification, Cleansing, Improved Environment

Nutrient Supplementation

H.O.P.E. Formula, Diet and Supplements

Awareness and Education

**MIDLINE**

Lack of Awareness

Poor Diet

Various Systemic Symptoms

Too Many Prescription Medications

Over Vaccination

Imbalanced Digestive Tract

Diabetes, Heart Disease, Arthritis, Inflammation

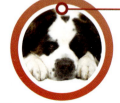

**CHRONIC HEALTH PROBLEMS**

(Figure 1)

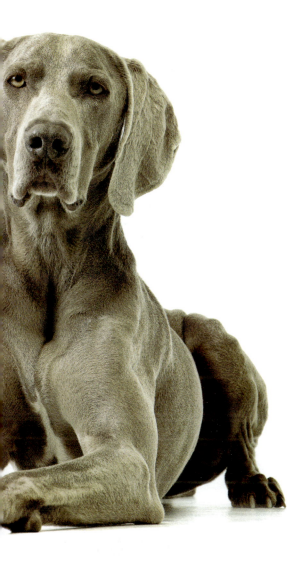

Dogs who are on the decline toward chronic health problems are usually in pain. Medications may alleviate obvious symptoms, but the jubilant wellness of your pet may not return as easily. Often owners will simply believe their dog is "getting older". Time after time, when you support and restore digestive health, overall vitality can be regained to any degree! The benefits of a lifelong natural maintenance/ prevention program can offer many years of health and happiness to your beloved pet, and save you a fortune in vet bills.

I realize that you may be completely overwhelmed with all of the options that are available to enhance canine health found in the local pet store or health food store. So, to simplify the choices, I'm going to explain why I highly recommend six options that are the foundation of nutritional health:

## H.O.P.E. and more:

**H.** **Higher-fiber** –(prebiotics) - a balance of soluble and insoluble fiber

**O.** **Omega-3 Oil** – essential fatty acids containing both EPA and DHA

**P.** **Probiotics** – containing at least 10 species of lactobacilli and bifidobacteria and at least 20 billion organisms per serving

**E.** **Enzymes** – Potent digestive enzymes formulated specifically to support the dietary needs of canines. These enzymes are needed to support the proper digestion of the protein, fat and carbohydrates found in a typical canine diet

**MORE** = **Nutraceuticals and Herbs**- there are many nutritional supplements and herbs that have very beneficial stress-relieving and anti-inflammatory properties for dogs.

## Vital Health

Health is a continuum, with optimal health at one end, and toxic overload, which may manifest as some form of disease or disability, or even cancer, at the opposite end. Optimal health, for both dogs and humans, is a dynamic process that is always moving in one direction or the other on this continuum (see figure 1).

A proactive approach is required to achieve optimal health regardless of where your dog's health is located on the continuum today. Pet parents who have dogs that seem to be in good health are less likely to believe or recognize how important it is to take preventive measures such as cleansing (detoxification) programs or adding digestive enzymes and/or probiotics to their dog's diet.

# TOP 3 REASONS WHY OUR PETS NEED SUPPLEMENTS?

**1. 90% OF PETS ARE FED DEAD FOOD!**

- Pet food that can sit in a can or a bag on the shelf for 2 years and not spoil is simply not living.

- Imagine eating nothing but the same processed food, every meal, everyday of your life. How would you feel?

- These foods only contain the minimum RDA of vitamins and minerals - **no living nutrients.**

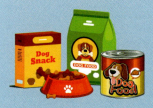

**2. PETS HAVE MORE TOXINS IN THEIR BODIES THAN WE DO!**

- Pets are lower to the ground and are exposed to more chemicals than we are.

- Pets lay on pet beds and furniture treated with fire retardant chemicals.

- Pets chew on plastic toys and get into various toxins in the trash, chemical waste, feces, etc.

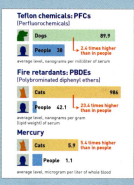

**Teflon chemicals: PFCs**
(Perfluorochemicals)

| | | |
|---|---|---|
| Dogs | | 89.9 |
| People | 38 | 2.4 times higher than in people |

average level, nanograms per milliliter of serum

**Fire retardants: PBDEs**
(Polybrominated diphenyl ethers)

| | | |
|---|---|---|
| Cats | | 986 |
| People | 42.1 | 23.4 times higher than in people |

average level, nanograms per gram (lipid weight) of serum

**Mercury**

| | | |
|---|---|---|
| Cats | 5.9 | 5.4 times higher than in people |
| People | 1.1 | |

average level, microgram per liter of whole blood

**3. DOGS & CATS HAVE COMPRESSED LIFESPANS!**

- Dogs and cats pack an entire life into an average of 13-15 years.

- The aging process is much more impactful on our pets.

- A dog or cat is the equivalent of human retirement age (63) by the time they reach their 9th birthday.

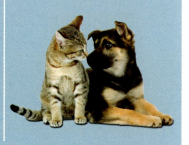

Responsible and informed choices for a healthy diet will offer your pet his greatest advantage for a long and happy life.

There is tremendous synergy when appropriate supplementation along with a healthy diet, are combined together to promote gastrointestinal health and thereby total body health.

Now let's take a look at why and how these components might be a good fit for your dog's unique situation.

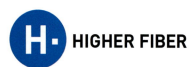

# HIGHER FIBER

## Fiber (Prebiotics)

Prebiotics are non-digestible food ingredients that beneficially affect your dog by promoting or stimulating the growth of good bacteria in the colon. The most common prebiotic is fiber,

and some types of fiber are fermented in the large intestine or colon. Fermentable fiber is beneficial for many reasons, including:

- Provides a source of energy for the cells of the colon to produce new cells

- Is essential for the healthy and balanced absorption of water from the colon

- Maintains healthy intestinal motility

- Inhibits the growth of pathogenic bacteria such as Clostridium or Salmonella

- Makes the colon cells healthier and more vigorous

- Reduces inflammation in the colon

- Creates a firmer stool

There are two main properties of fiber that vary in ratio to each other known as "soluble" and "insoluble". The soluble part in particular offers many benefits for daily intestinal health. Acacia is one of the best sources of primarily soluble fiber, and it is also one of the most naturally fermentable fibers, which makes it an excellent prebiotic.

**The soluble portion of fiber:**

- Promotes the growth of probiotics by acting as a food for the good bacteria
- Slows the rate of carbohydrate absorption
- Promotes healthy blood sugar and insulin metabolism
- Helps normalize appetite
- Decreases LDL (bad cholesterol) levels
- Helps eliminate toxins from the body
- Supports healthy kidney function

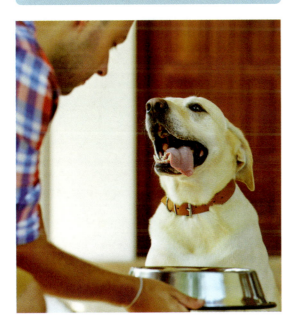

The "soluble" in soluble fiber means that it dissolves in water (though it is not digested). This allows it to absorb excess liquid in the colon, preventing the onset of diarrhea by adding necessary bulk to the stool and forming a thick gel to lubricate the bowel. This gel (as opposed to a watery liquid) also keeps the GI muscles stretched gently around a full colon, giving those muscles something to easily "grip" during the peristaltic contractions and thus preventing the rapid transit time and

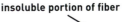
insoluble portion of fiber

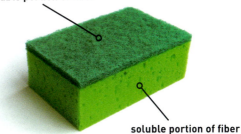
soluble portion of fiber

explosive bowel movements associated with diarrhea. Since diarrhea can be an important symptom of a serious health condition, if your dog is suffering from watery stool diarrhea, it's time for a visit to your vet. However, many dogs experience soft stools on a chronic basis and relief for both you and your pet may be experienced simply by adding fiber to her diet.

**The insoluble portion of fiber:**

- Sweeps clean the digestive tract
- Helps eliminate toxins
- Tones the bowel by creating volume, giving the muscles exercise
- Increases peristalsis, the muscle motion necessary for healthy elimination

Since insoluble fibers are not digested at all, they pass through the gut essentially unchanged. **Insoluble fiber can help dogs lose or maintain healthy body weight by increasing the volume of food they can eat without adding much in the way of calories**. Since insoluble fiber also adds bulk to the stool which stimulates movement within the intestinal tract, it can be helpful in some cases of canine constipation, as well as with diarrhea (discussed above).

**Another positive side effect of fiber is that the added bulk in the stool helps your pet empty the glands located in the anal sphincter. Anal glands in dogs often get diseased and impacted, which may result in pain and rectal abscess**. A very common symptom of a full anal gland is the "floor-scooting" motion our dogs sometimes demonstrate.

# BRENDA'S POOP SCOOP

## HEALTHY DOGGY POOP

### COLOR WHEEL

Your dog's stool should be chocolate brown. Consuming different foods can cause some color variations. For example, veggies like beet, carrots or greens can color the stool.

### SHAPE

Your dog's poop should be a somewhat oblong shape. It could even look like a small version of a cow patty or a banana. If you are feeding a raw food diet, the poop could be small, hard balls, easily passed that degrade in the yard quickly. This is normal poop for a raw-fed dog.

### CONSISTENCY

A normal bowel movement should feel be a bit like putty as you put it into the doggy bag. However, it shouldn't melt into the grass as you pick it up. Hard stool could indicate dehydration. Loose stool can indicate an issue as simple as your dog eating something rotten on the path or other more serious intestinal issues. Call your vet if diarrhea is persistent.

### SIZE

2 things can affect the amount of your dog's poop. 1. How much food he/she consumes and 2. How much fiber is in the food. Fiber is a very good thing and it is always better to have more healthy stool than less. With a raw food diet, you may notice less volume of stool.

### CONTENT

Mucus in the stool indicates inflammation in the intestine. Grass in the stool may be the result of gastric upset or stress. Hair in the stool could reflect a skin condition.

## POOP COLORS

Changes in color of your dog's stool could indicate internal issues. Consult your vet to be sure the poop is healthy.

**WHITE GRAINS**
could indicate tapeworm

**GREY/GREASY**
could indicate pancreas or bile issue

**BLACK/TARRY**
could indicate bleeding in the upper digestive system

**BRIGHT RED STREAKS**
could indicate blood in stool. Check your dog for rectal bleeding or cuts

**ORANGE/YELLOW**
could be a bile or liver issue

**GREEN**
could be your dog is eating a lot of grass. Could also indicate a gall bladder problem

**CHOCOLATE BROWN**
Normal

## BRENDA'S FUN POOP Q & A

**Q: How many bowel movements are normal for my dog daily?**
**A:** At least one, and two or three is not unusual.

**Suggestion:** Please recognize that more poop is in most cases a sign your dog's digestive system is working effectively. Buy more poop bags!

**Q: Why does my dog eat poop?**
**A:** The truth is, no one knows for sure. One thought is that they are seeking additional nutrients or specific bacteria. I have 4 dogs, and one eats poop. The crazy thing is that my poop-eater will only eat the poop of a certain one of my other 3 dogs!

**Suggestion:** Start your pet on a good probiotic! Often that will do the trick.

**Q: Why is my dog scooting on his behind?**
**A:** Dogs scoot on their butts often when they are experiencing diarrhea. It's their attempt to find toilet paper. If the stool is normal, it's possible that your pet has irritating impacted anal glands.

**Suggestion:** Increase the fiber in your dog's diet. Not only will this provide a more formed stool, but fiber also exercises the colon and massages the anal glands.

**Q: Why does it seem that every time I change my dog's diet, his poop changes?**
**A:** Just like with your own diet, changing the foods you eat often has an effect on your own bowel movements. By the way, a more diverse diet is actually good for a healthy dog (and a healthy person).

**Suggestion:** Give the new diet a few days and see if the poop normalizes. Often it will. Remember, if you have decided to offer a raw food diet, your dog's poop will be different than when fed a standard commercially produced product. Good news – it will be less smelly!

## DR. MURPHY

Dietary fiber is divided into 2 groups - soluble and insoluble fiber. Insoluble fiber can be very beneficial for dogs that suffer from anal gland issues. Soluble fiber is the primary fiber we are interested in for improving a dog's health. Soluble fiber helps create the right environment in the colon for healthy bacteria. This is why it is referred to as a prebiotic. Often dogs with chronic colitis or sensitive colons that are prone to diarrhea benefit from increasing soluble fiber in the diet.

As a caring pet parent, monitoring your dog's poop habits are extremely helpful in determining overall wellness. Let's face it, picking up a well-formed stool is a much more pleasant task for you, and is a great indicator of good intestinal health in your dog.

SPECIFICALLY, THERE ARE TWO WAYS FIBER CAN BE EXTREMELY HELPFUL FOR BOTH OVERWEIGHT DOGS AND ONES DIAGNOSED WITH DIABETES.

1. FIBER HELPS YOUR DOG FEEL FULL AND WILL HELP HIM TO EAT LESS

2. FIBER SLOWS THE ENTRANCE OF GLUCOSE INTO THE BLOODSTREAM

## 5 MOST COMMON DIABETES SYMPTOMS IN DOGS:

## INCREASED THIRST

## INCREASED URINATION

## INCREASED HUNGER WHILE LOSING WEIGHT

## LOWER ACTIVITY

## THINNING, DRY, OR DULL HAIR

## CLOUDY EYES

Higher fiber becomes absolutely essential if your dog's diet has a relatively high carbohydrate or fat content that potentially could result in diabetes or high cholesterol. It's also important to note that certain breeds have a genetic disposition to these conditions, so overall, once again, prevention is central to ensuring your dog's well-being long term. Stay with me and I promise this will become even clearer in a future chapter.

### TIP

### CHOOSING THE BEST FIBER

Look for a product that contains both soluble and insoluble fibers. Products offering combinations of excellent sources of fiber for your dog may include:

- Acacia fiber
- Apple pectin
- Pumpkin
- Flax

Often these products will be available as a powder that is easy to scoop onto your dog's daily meals.

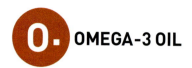

# O. OMEGA-3 OIL

Essential fatty acids (EFAs) are required for the proper structure and function of every cell in the body. In the wild, a dog would glean his EFAs from meat sources primarily. Omega-3 and omega-6 oils are both types of essential fatty acids.

### Omega-3 Fatty Acids

Of all the nutritional supplements that reduce inflammation in dogs as well as humans, none has been researched as intensely as omega-3 fatty acids. Research has shown that these essential fatty acids are effective in reducing inflammation in dogs with allergic dermatitis. Their anti-inflammatory effects are beneficial not just for skin conditions, but for kidney disease, heart disease and joint disease as well.

## TOO MANY OMEGA-6 FATTY ACIDS ACTUALLY INCREASE SKIN INFLAMMATION FROM ALLERGIES. SOME SOURCES OF OMEGA-6S ARE:

## GRAINS

## LEGUMES

## VEGETABLE OILS (CORN, SUNFLOWER, SOYBEAN)

## EGGS

Dogs are designed to use and process the fat in their diets differently than the human body does. For example, they naturally have more good cholesterol (HDL) than bad cholesterol (LDL). A dog or cat won't develop high blood cholesterol or thickening of the arteries from fat in the diet. Generally, fats aren't considered to be bad for your dog's health except in the case where obese dogs are fed diets high in both fat and calories (often from too many carbohydrates).

Omega-6 fatty acids have the opposite effect of omega-3 fats and too many omega-6s increase inflammation. Canine diets tend to be very high in omega-6 because of all the legume and grain ingredients found in commercial dog foods, whereas in the wild, dogs typically consume far less omega-6 fatty acids.

**TIP**

**Omega-3 fatty acids decrease inflammation**

**Omega-6 fatty acids increase inflammation**

Omega-6 fatty acids are often added to canine diets because they make the dog's coat look shiny and glossy, but most pet owners don't realize that the benefit of a shiny coat comes at the expense of increased inflammation. So how do we safely give our dogs a lustrous and shiny coat without increasing the internal inflammatory response? A better choice is safer omega-6 fatty acids such as gamma-linoleic acid (GLA) found in primrose oil, borage oil and black currant seed oil, but these oils are very expensive and not found in dog foods.

While nutritional supplementation on its own does not provide an alternative to corticosteroid in dogs with severe allergies, shortly you will find out that the right supplements can greatly reduce the amount of medication needed and often reduces the side effects of drug therapy.

## DR. MURPHY

The biggest problem with omega-3 and omega-6 fatty acids included in dog food is that they easily become rancid and unhealthy for dogs. Omega 3 fatty acids become rancid and harmful even more quickly than omega-6s.

## DR. MURPHY

When a dog is miserable with persistent itching, unable to sleep, and even mutilating his body, corticosteroid therapy is necessary. In severe allergies dogs can literally chew their skin off. Unfortunately, corticosteroids have side effects, so veterinarians are usually careful to use the lowest dose of corticosteroids and for the shortest amount of time to minimize potential side effects. Newer veterinary medicines that target kinases and interleukins can also reduce or eliminate the need for cortisone. These drugs like all drugs have side effects but generally less than corticosteroids.

Interestingly, a food allergy in a dog does not respond very well to corticosteroids. So, when itching does not abate with cortisone therapy, veterinarians start looking for less common allergies like food allergy, contact allergy, drug reactions or parasites in the skin like scabies.

About 15-20% of dogs with atopic dermatitis can be controlled with omega- 3 fatty acid therapy, flea control, and supplements. While these holistic approaches will not stop itching in 100% of dogs, 80% of dogs will respond positively to more natural treatments and the veterinarian can greatly reduce the dosage of drugs needed to control the allergy.

Since the short and long-term effects of corticosteroids are greatly affected by the amount and duration of cortisone given, any reduction in these necessary drugs can hugely benefit the overall health of your dog.

## DR. MURPHY

### How much omega-3 does your pet need to reduce inflammation?

At least 600 mg of omega-3 fatty acids. In practice, I have found that omega-3 fatty acids need to be given daily for at least two months before clinical signs of reduced inflammation can be observed in dogs. Omega-3 fatty acids are very beneficial in controlling inflammation in the skin caused by allergies, and in many cases omega-3s combined with herbal and nutritional therapies are effective in controlling and relieving allergic dermatitis in dogs.

Omega-3 fatty acids support the functions of joint and connective tissue. Additionally, omega fatty acids are vital to everyday health and strong muscles. Omega-3 fatty acids are multi-purpose supplements and serve as an excellent adjunctive support in many inflammatory conditions.

### Omega-3 fatty acids

- Are very beneficial for cognitive dysfunction in dogs
- Aid in the proper development of the retina and visual cortex
- Regulate blood-clotting activity
- Slow the development and spread of certain pet cancers
- Reduce amount of NSAIDS needed for treatment of osteoarthritis
- Treat and slow the progression of kidney disease
- Give pets getting chemotherapy longer survival times
- Help in treatment of epilepsy refractory to antiepileptic drug therapy
- Help support dogs with muscle weight loss from heart failure

Another inflammatory condition that pet parent's encounter are hip and joint issues. While there are many approaches to managing hip and joint discomfort in dogs, a majority of vets utilize a combination of prescription medication, diet and lifestyle changes, including natural remedies such as herbal therapy and supplements.

**TIP**

## HOW TO CHOOSE THE BEST OMEGA-3 SUPPLEMENT

Dogs need a relatively high level of supplemental omega-3s to be effective since most commercial foods don't adequately provide this important nutrient. For this reason, choosing a quality omega-3 formula is critical.

Look for a fish oil supplement that contains at least 600mg of omega-3 per soft gel. Some soft gel formulas even include a delicious flavor on the outside of the gel for ease of use. Many dog foods mention omega-3 on the label but include only a tiny amount simply for marketing and advertising purposes. Plus, these oils start to oxidize and turn rancid when they are exposed to oxygen during the manufacturing process. Please don't be fooled, for your dog's sake.

Choosing a quality source of omega 3 is very important. Omega-3 oils from large fish like salmon are usually highly contaminated with dioxins, PCPs,

mercury, heavy metals, and other toxins. The best fish sources would be smaller fish like anchovies, sardines, mackerel and/or herring which don't accumulate toxins as readily.

Plant oils like flax seed oil contain ALA (alpha-linolenic acid) which, through a conversion process in the body, can be broken down to omega-3 fatty acids. However, dogs do not convert ALA to omega-3 fatty acids very well. Plant based oils such as flax seed oil are simply not as useful as an omega-3 supplement derived from fish oil for your dog. In fact, fish oil is far superior to flax seed oil when supplementing for purposes of decreasing inflammatory processes.

When choosing the right omega-3 for your pet, be sure that the fish oil has been purified to remove any toxins, and that this is stated clearly on the label. Look for certification by a 3rd party certifier that tests the oils for potency and purity. If the oil hasn't been purified, your pet could be getting contaminants like mercury which can damage the nervous system over time.

## P. PROBIOTICS

Your dog's intestinal tract normally contains upwards of 500 different species of bacteria, perhaps as many as 1,000. As you now understand, good bacteria are critical to good health and the immune system, and a diverse bacterial community is a strong indicator of a healthy dog.

The term "probiotics" comes from the Greek words "pro" and "biotics," meaning "for life" or "in favor of life" respectively. It's a high priority that the right ratio of good bacteria to bad bacteria be maintained in your dog's intestine. Always remember that up to 80% of your dog's immune defenses are located in the digestive tract.

As you've learned, imbalance of gut flora is the second step in the Process of Declining Health, leading to intestinal toxemia, and beyond. Balancing gut bacteria is not only important to re-establishing a healthy balance for your dog's gut, but also critical in maintaining digestive health and overall vitality throughout his entire life.

We've talked a lot about pathogenic bacteria, parasites and other bad guys. Now let's focus in on the good bacteria – what they are and how we can make sure to support our pet's health with the good guys.

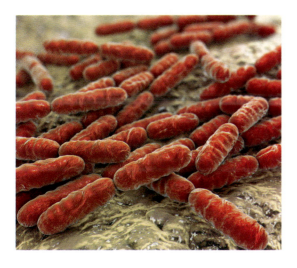

### Benefits Probiotics Provide to Your Dog's Health

Probiotics directly affect many areas of a dog's digestive system including his mouth, esophagus, stomach, small and large intestines. It's impossible to list all the positive functions that probiotics accomplish for your dog's well-being. New and valuable functions are discovered almost daily in research. Let me share with you just a few positive actions that probiotics perform here:

- Assist in the digestion and absorption of essential nutrients
- Support his immune system
- Support the intestinal environment to promote proper digestion
- Help maintain healthy bowel function
- Nourish and balance natural gut bacteria

### Replacing Probiotics in Your Dog's Digestive Tract

In order to balance gut flora, we can easily and effectively return the good bacteria to the digestive tract with a probiotic formula.

Probiotics are predominately bacterial; however, some fungi (like Saccharomyces boulardii) are also considered beneficial "probiotic" microorganisms.

### Resident vs. Transient Strains

Another important point about good bacteria involves the relationship between resident and transient strains. Resident strains are those strains that are commonly found in your dog's digestive tract. Lactobacillus acidophilus and Bifidobacterium bifidum are common resident strains found virtually in all dog's intestinal systems. Lactobacillus casei, Lactobacillus bulgarius and Streptococcus thermophillus are

## DR. MURPHY

Your dog's body just like our body is the host for trillions of bacteria. These are called the animal's microbiota. The health of these trillions of bacteria are linked in vibrant health or the advent of disease in your dog. You cannot separate the dog's body from the microbiota. They are completely dependent on each other.

You can support and heal your dog's microbiota by infusing healthy bacteria and providing insoluble fiber that enhances the well-being of the microbiota. Probiotics can stimulate the immune system, buffer and block the effects of unhealthy bacteria, treat diarrhea, even reduce flatulence. Current research is indicating far reaching effects on the overall health of the body, from reduction in duration of respiratory infections to positive effects on the neurological system and central nervous system, to name just a few.

As a holistic veterinarian, I believe that probiotics and prebiotics are foundational for maintaining a dog's vitality and offering your pet the best opportunity for longevity.

stimulating the growth and/or activity of one or a limited number of bacteria in the colon" (Gibson and Roberfroid, 1995). We've discussed fiber as a prebiotic.

A prebiotic is further defined as a dietary ingredient that reaches the large intestine in an intact form and has a specific metabolic function supporting beneficial rather than harmful bacteria. A true prebiotic must:

1. Be neither hydrolyzed nor absorbed by the upper part of the digestive tract

2. Be a surface on which an organism can grow for one or a limited number of beneficial bacteria

3. Be able to help restore the appropriate 80:20 bacterial balance

4. Offer healing effects to the intestinal lining and/or other area of your dog's body

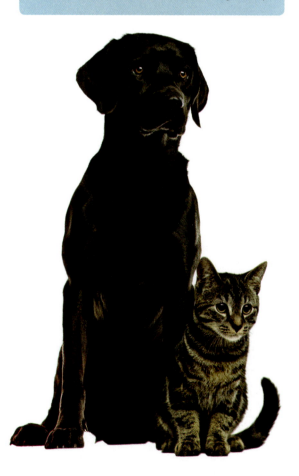

common transient strains. Transient strains are often found in foods like kefir. These strains will not take up residence in your dog's digestive tract; however, they do provide many benefits as they pass through.

## Probiotics and Prebiotics

Probiotics have been defined as living microorganisms that improve health and balance the intestinal environment. A prebiotic is defined as "a non-digestible food ingredient that beneficially affects the host by selectively

## SELECTING THE BEST PROBIOTIC FOR YOUR DOG

There are many companies offering probiotic products for dogs today. Each probiotic formula will be different. The products will have different types of strains and numbers of cultures; they may or may not be packaged with a prebiotic, and they will have a broad range of prices. In order to make a selection, consider the following:

**High Potency:** A minimum of 20 billion live cultures per serving. Since there are billions of bacteria in your dog's digestive tract it is important that a probiotic supplement provide a sufficient dose of the friendly bacteria.

**Multi-Strain:** A minimum of 10 unique strains (different kinds) of bacteria. A proper blend should include Lactobacillus and Bifidobacterium strains. A probiotic supplement should contain a blend of clinically studied animal strains such as B. animalis. Many probiotic supplements contain just 1 or 2 strains of good bacteria.

**GMP Certification:** Good Manufacturing Practices ensure that a supplement contains what is claimed on its label and is manufactured using the highest quality standards.

**Prebiotics:** Serve as food for the beneficial bacteria to help them multiply and survive.

Our dog's health is precious! They provide us with unconditional love and companionship. A daily probiotic formula is a great way to ensure good health. Make sure you choose one that delivers the recommended potency level and strain count. There is nothing quite like a healthy and happy dog. Happy Dog, Happy Life!

# E. ENZYME SUPPORT

As you learned in Chapter 1, enzymes are essential for all chemical processes in the body, including digestion.

We discussed previously that dogs don't produce a lot of enzymes for carbohydrate digestion because their natural, ancestral diet is primarily meat (protein & fat) -- not grains (carbs).

Your dog's pancreas, which manufactures amylase to breakdown carbohydrates, simply cannot secrete enough digestive enzymes to do so effectively - considering the large amount of carbohydrates that are present in commercial dog foods.

It's very interesting to recognize that your pets were designed to get some supplemental enzymes from the foods they eat. When wolves and coyotes hunt and kill animals in the wild they eat some of the entrails, "the guts", to meet their digestive enzyme needs.

Of course, we typically don't feed our dogs and cats those innards they'd be getting in the wild. The sad result is that most pets in the United States can easily be enzyme-deficient.

## IMPORTANT NOTE
### THE ENZYMES CONTAINED IN RAW FOODS ONLY BREAK DOWN THE FOODS THEY'RE CONTAINED WITHIN. THEY DON'T HELP DIGEST OTHER DEAD FOODS THAT MAY BE CONSUMED IN THE MEAL.

## DR. MURPHY

Throughout history dogs have evolved as hunters and scavengers and their digestive systems adapted to eating the organ meats of their prey raw, including the prey's pancreas. In fact, in nature, a wolf or wild dog will actually eat the organs first, ingesting valuable enzymes in the process.

Modern pet dogs are fed highly processed grains, skeletal meat with additives and processed foods not found prior to our commercial society, not to mention the genetically modified foods (GMOs).

An important question holistic veterinarians ask as they encounter modern health issues is this - is the dog's pancreas and intestinal mucosa up to the enzymatic challenge of their modern diet?

In most patients we see the benefit to giving additional digestive enzymes result in better formed stool, reduced vomiting and even reduced diarrhea. These are just the easily observable benefits.

Better digestion means healthier intestinal mucosa and better absorption and assimilation of nutrients. Reducing the volume of incompletely digested foods that the immune system and liver have to deal with reduces the drain on your dog's vital energy and overall health. Poorly digested food upsets your dog's natural intestinal bacteria and can cause the gastrointestinal upsets I mentioned such as vomiting and diarrhea and over time leads to chronic disease.

When you consider your dog's health, why would you not give your pet additional enzymes?

Raw meat and vegetables contain live enzymes that can greatly help your pet's digestive process, however those valuable enzymes are killed with heat.

Canned dog food and dry kibble have been cooked and are completely devoid of any enzymes.

What this means is that your pet could be lacking in the enzymes it needs to digest its food properly. This puts extreme stress on his digestive system, which can ultimately interfere with nutrient absorption and cause recurrent digestive issues and declining health.

Supplementing with digestive enzymes will decrease the stress on the pancreas, increase digestive functionality and support your dog's immune system.

**A good digestive enzyme formula will contain a variety of enzymes:**

- Amylase aids in digestion of carbohydrates
- Protease aids in digestion of proteins
- Lipase aids in digestion of fats

As enzyme reserves become depleted, it can lead to a range of health issues in your pet that we discussed in chapter 2, not to mention malabsorption of nutrients and improper food digestion.

In a future chapter we will discuss realistic options for dietary support. In the majority of situations when you are purchasing foods from a store, your dog will most likely benefit from enzyme supplementation.

## TIP

### CHOOSING THE BEST ENZYME SUPPORT FOR YOUR DOG

In searching for a digestive enzyme for your pet, look for one that is in a powdered form, easy to sprinkle on your dog's food.

Look for a product that contains a powerful digestive enzyme blend that has been formulated specifically to support the dietary needs of canines. It's important that it contains protease, amylase and lipase to digest the major nutritional components found in a healthy canine diet.

Some combination formulas out there will combine digestive enzymes with other ingredients known to support proper digestive health such as organic pumpkin, fennel and ginger.

To recap, whether your pet is young and seemingly healthy or already experiencing digestive issues, supplementing with digestive enzymes is an easy and inexpensive way to know that your dog is processing his food more completely, giving him the extra support to live more years with ease and happiness. Be proactive and start now!

WHEN DIGESTION IS INCOMPLETE, PLANT ENZYMES ACT LIKE "PAC MAN,™" BREAKING DOWN AND CLEANING UP UNDIGESTED FOOD IN THE DIGESTIVE TRACT. **WHEN NOT FULLY DIGESTED, THIS FOOD CAN GIVE RISE TO INTESTINAL TOXEMIA, AND ULTIMATELY, TOXIC OVERLOAD.**

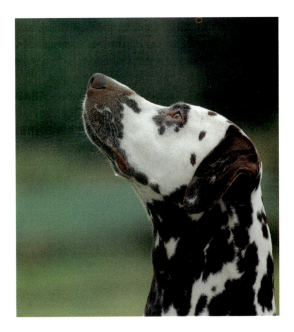

# MORE

## NUTRACEUTICALS AND HERBS

Our loving dogs depend on us to provide them with the building blocks of health, from quality foods to daily exercise to targeted supplements. As thoughtful and responsible caregivers, we have the opportunity to make choices that can proactively improve the quality of life of our companion animals. Let's take a look at a few nutraceuticals (an ingredient that provides a health benefit) and herbs you may find blended together in products at your favorite pet or health food store.

### Anxiety and Stress

For calming purposes like separation anxiety, thunderstorms, car rides, rehabilitation from injury and other situations that may disturb the peace of your pet look for a product containing:

**GABA** – a neurotransmitter in your pet's central nervous system. Research has found that too little GABA in the nervous system can contribute to feelings of panic and anxiety. GABA can promote a calming effect on nerves.

**L-Theanine** – is an amino acid derived from tea that helps maintain immunity and may help relieve anxiety and tension. It also supports healthy brain and nerve function.

**Chamomile** – one of the most popular herbs in the western world. Chamomile has a long history of promoting a sense of relaxation without a strong sedative effect. It helps to mitigate the "fight or flight" response that can cause overstimulation.

**Valerian root** – used as an herbal sleep aid since the times of Ancient Greece. In small amounts, it can help reduce the effects of normal environmental stress.

**Lemon balm** – used since the Middle Ages as a support for anxiety, irritability and tension. It has been shown to help promote a sound and restful sleep.

**Flower essences** – pure vibrational therapies from nature. They work at the subtle level of thoughts and emotions. Flower essences are one of the most effective therapies we have for supporting normal emotional balance of our pets.

The above remedies when synergistically combined in a supplement form are very effective at helping to calm dogs exhibiting nervousness, hyperactivity, discontentment or responding to environmentally-induced stress.

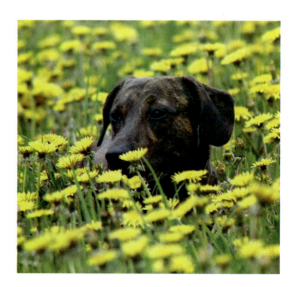

## DR. MURPHY

Flower essences are unique vibrational therapies that affect the quantum informational field (the part that resides in the dimension of thought in physics). They have been shown for decades to help heal the immune system and balance the body's bio-energy fields. A balanced bio-energy field is resistant to disease and allergic reactions. As we discussed in Chapter 2, stress and anxiety negatively impact immune system functions, as well as digestion.

Used as a holistic healing therapy since the 1920s, the unique aspects of these natural vibrational therapies make them very safe. A dog can never overdose on flower essences or be harmed by using the "wrong" flower essence. The body takes only the vibrational therapy that it needs.

Flower essences are not aromatherapy or fragrant. The term flower essences may conjure up thoughts of sweet fragrances, but flower essences actually have no scent at all and should not be confused with aromatherapy or essential oils.

Flower essences are also not herbs or drugs, which have their effects on the physical body. Instead they work on the dimension of thought, strengthening a healthy mind-body link. They do not interfere or interact with any drugs, surgery or herbal medications. Although similar to homeopathic remedies, flower essences work more deeply and are often considered even safer than homeopathic remedies.

## Hip, Joint, Arthritis and Inflammatory Conditions

For anti-inflammatory purposes like soreness upon movement, and hip and joint disorders look for a product containing:

**Glucosamine** – a natural compound found in healthy cartilage. Glucosamine is commonly taken in combination with chondroitin, which supports healthy connective tissue.

**Boswellia** – used for centuries to support hip and joint health

**Green-Lipped Mussel** – a natural source of rich Omega-3 fatty acids

**Turmeric** – has strong anti-inflammatory and antioxidant properties. It's beneficial constituent, curcumin is responsible for the bright yellow color of turmeric and is believed to be the principal active agent.

**MSM** – considered a building block for cartilage repair. MSM contains glycosaminoglycans that enable cartilage to soak up water and thus act as a cushion for bones.

**Flower essences** – work on a subatomic vibrational level. Some formulas on the market contain exclusive flower essences blends created specifically to support joint function.

> **TIP** Omega-3 oils are always a great addition to any anti-inflammatory protocol!

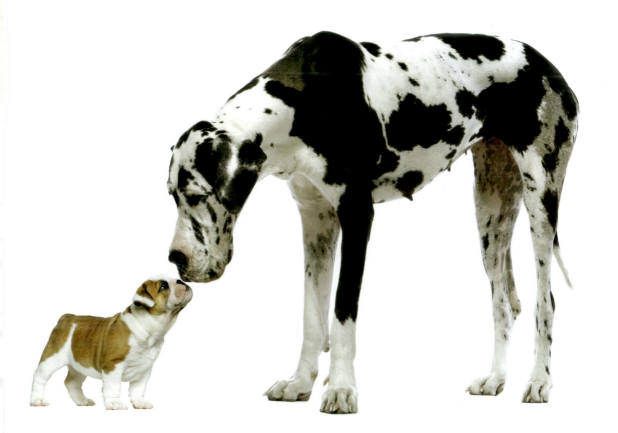

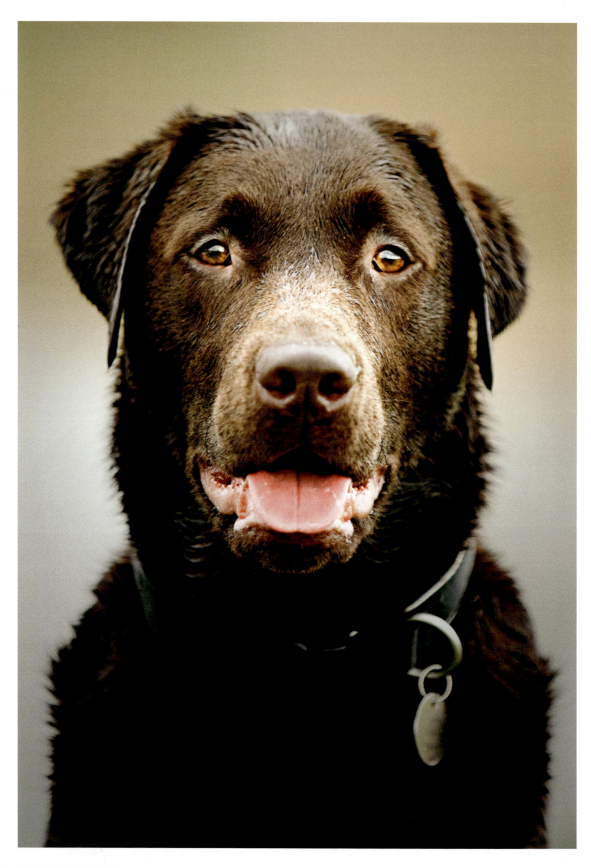

CHAPTER 5

# CHOOSING THE BEST FOOD FOR YOUR BEST FRIEND (AND FOR YOU, TOO!)

Ultimately, my goal in writing this book is to help concerned pet parents really understand what they can do to enjoy the maximum number of years with their best four-legged friend while keeping him or her happy and vital! The information I've presented is tremendously important to me personally, as I have four dogs myself, ranging in ages between 1 and 11 years old.

Throughout my entire career I've been teaching about gut health in humans. Most of the physiological processes are similar in dogs and humans. However, the nutritional needs of your pet are distinctly different from yours. Just as in humans, central to their vitality and longevity is the nutrition your dog is offered daily.

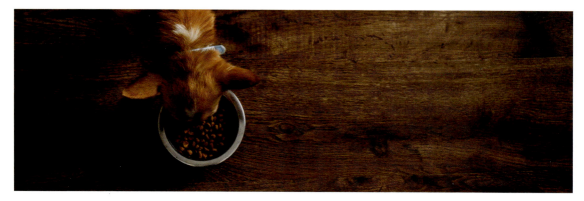

Have you ever stood in the pet food aisle or pet store and found yourself completely overwhelmed? I know I have. Perhaps you finally grab a bag of dog food that has images of beautiful meats and veggies on the front, possibly with a picture of a well-known personality, a gorgeous wild wolf, or even a picture of your very own breed of dog, clearly in perfect and vigorous health.

I'm certain that everyone reading this book wants to be the very best pet parent they can possibly be. I know I do! Truth is, dietary choices for your dog actually present some unique challenges for us and may impact important factors in our own lives.

After all, wouldn't we all like to provide for ourselves and our families freshly prepared organic non-GMO meals with grass-fed meats – and then the factors of life step in! Don't despair! After reading this chapter, I hope I will have offered you a workable solution to improve your pet's health, no matter what dog food choice you make, one step at a time.

Many of you at this point may be feeding commercial dog food (kibble and/or canned). Convenience, price, and confusion may be the reason. Any food that is AAFCO-approved, meaning it contains a certain compliment of vitamins and minerals will certainly keep your dog alive. Unfortunately, it is not the best way for your pet to thrive.

**As I offer dietary options for your best friend, I am committed to considering the following factors for both you and me:**

**Time:**

- How much time do I have to prepare my dog's food?

- If I am going to make my pet's food, am I disciplined enough to faithfully follow a recipe made by a PhD in pet nutrition so that my pet gets a balanced diet?

**Availability:**

- How available am I to create a regular feeding schedule for my dog, considering my work schedule and time commitments?

**Finances:**

- How much money can I responsibly spend on my pet's food?

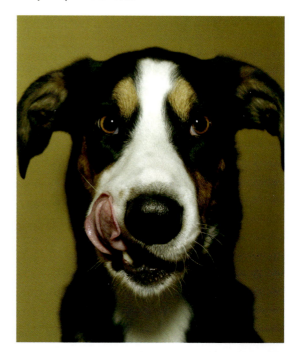

**Here's a short reminder list of why many commercial pet foods are not optimal nutrition for your dog:**

• The food itself is "dead" due to how it must be processed (the technical term is "extruded") in order to be packaged or canned. Heat completely destroys all the vital nutrients available in fresh food like good bacteria, enzymes and omega-3 oils.

• Preservatives are regularly added to the foods in order for them to remain on the store shelves for extended periods of time. Examples of preservatives are BHA, BHT and ethoxygin. Without these preservatives fungus (mold) such as aspergillus can grow and release dangerous aflatoxins in the food that can cause death, cancer, liver and kidney disease. The only way to avoid using preservatives in food is by high quality canning methods, refrigeration or freezing.

• The extremely high heat required by the commercial processes discussed in chapter 2 create known carcinogens like acrylamide from carbohydrates and heterocyclic amines from proteins.

• Most kibble products, treats and even many canned foods are heavily laden with unnecessary carbohydrates for your dog that promote "age-related" disorders like obesity, arthritis and diabetes, just to name a few.

• And last, but definitely not least – kibble has only approximately 12% moisture content! Your dog's ancestral diet provided around 70% moisture on a daily basis. Too often the foods we serve are slowly but surely creating low-grade dehydration throughout our pet's life!

**Check out the Resources section for more info on these topics**.

## THE MOISTURE CONTENT OF FOOD
## MAY BE THE SINGLE MOST IMPORTANT CONSIDERATION FOR YOUR DOG'S LONG-TERM HEALTH AND VITALITY!

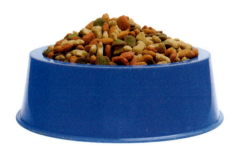

In order to make informed feeding decisions, it's important to understand what's available on the market. So I'd like to offer a general overview on some possible food choices for your dog – from best to worst - both from a quality and a situational standpoint. Truly, it would take an entire book to adequately cover this subject.

**Much more detailed information on this subject is available through authorities I'm offering in the Resources section of this book**.

Please don't be dismayed. Just because you may not be able to provide the #1 choice consistently doesn't mean you can't offer your dog great food to fulfill optimum nutritional needs, considering your lifestyle factors. Personally, I make about three homemade meals for my dogs weekly. As we continue I promise to share suggestions that can satisfy both of you and maintain your dear pet's health!

Good news! There is intense demand from dog owners for healthy food for their pets. This consumer demand for safe and healthy food has forced the dog food companies to make better and better foods to compete in a very crowded marketplace. A bit of research into the company that manufactures the food will provide both quality food for your dog and peace of mind for you. More expensive is not always better.

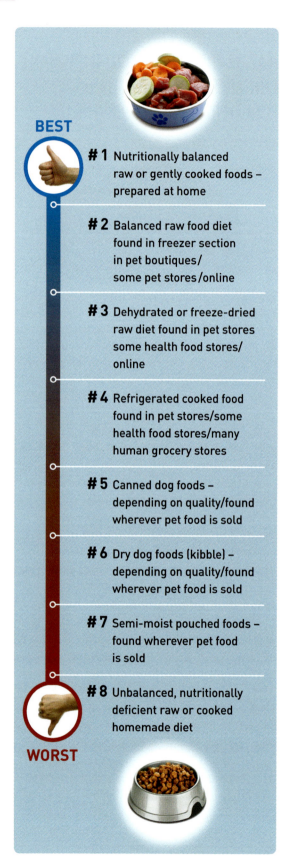

**BEST**

**#1** Nutritionally balanced raw or gently cooked foods – prepared at home

**#2** Balanced raw food diet found in freezer section in pet boutiques/ some pet stores/online

**#3** Dehydrated or freeze-dried raw diet found in pet stores some health food stores/ online

**#4** Refrigerated cooked food found in pet stores/some health food stores/many human grocery stores

**#5** Canned dog foods – depending on quality/found wherever pet food is sold

**#6** Dry dog foods (kibble) – depending on quality/found wherever pet food is sold

**#7** Semi-moist pouched foods – found wherever pet food is sold

**#8** Unbalanced, nutritionally deficient raw or cooked homemade diet

**WORST**

I'd like to offer a brief discussion of the pros and cons of each category of food for your consideration:

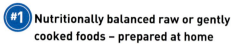

**#1** **Nutritionally balanced raw or gently cooked foods – prepared at home**

**Pros:**

- Biologically appropriate when prepared properly

- Benefits of a raw food diet are reported as:
  - shinier coats
  - healthier skin
  - cleaner teeth
  - higher energy
  - smaller stools

- You can choose all the ingredients and know exactly what your dog is eating.

- Moisture rich, especially raw offerings and foods gently cooked at lower temperatures

**Cons:**

- Time consuming preparation

- A proper education is absolutely necessary for the pet guardian in order to prepare and provide a nutritionally complete diet offering appropriate vitamin and mineral content.

- May be expensive, depending on the quality of ingredients chosen

- Someone must be available to feed your dog twice daily.

- Potential health threat due to bacteria in raw meat and possibility of improper storage. Food cannot be left out uneaten or it will spoil.

- Whole bones could choke or break teeth, depending on the age and breed of your dog. Again, proper education is critical.

- Some dogs prefer cooked food over raw.

**Suggestions for improvement:**
Even with the very best diet plans, adding in probiotics and digestive enzymes will support healthy digestion.

**TIP**

**#2** **Balanced raw food diet. Found in freezer section in pet boutiques/some pet stores /online**

**Pros:**

- More convenient than raw food prepared at home – saves time for pet guardian.

- If AAFCO compliant and labeled as "nutritionally balanced for all life stages", frozen raw food may afford similar benefits to raw food prepared at home.

**TIP**

The best raw frozen foods will be formulated on a caloric basis and on the label, the protein, fat, and other nutrients will be expressed as grams or milligrams per 1000 kcal. If on the label, the protein is expressed as a percentage (ex: crude protein – 20%) this indicates the product was formulated on a dry matter basis and will be significantly lower in nutrients. Bottom line, if you're going to spend the money on frozen raw foods, choose the product that is formulated on a caloric basis.

**Cons:**

- Relatively expensive

- Requires freezer space

- Proper storage is essential. Food cannot be left out uneaten.

- Someone must be available to feed your dog twice daily.

**TIP**

**Suggestions for improvement:**
As with raw and gently cooked foods, adding in probiotics and digestive enzymes will always support healthy digestion.

**#3** **Dehydrated or freeze-dried raw diet. Found in pet stores/some health food stores/online**

**Pros:**

- Very good nutrient value (minus a balanced fatty acid profile) due to low heat processing

- Shelf stable – doesn't require refrigeration

- Extremely convenient – just add water

- Excellent moisture content due to addition of water in preparation

**Cons:**

- Research of company is imperative to determine quality of ingredients.

- If you intend to regularly feed these products, be sure the label reads "AAFCO-approved and nutritionally balanced for all life stages".

- If the label reads "for supplemental feeding" do not use this as a primary nutrient source for your pet, however it can be an easy and healthful supplement to your dog's weekly diet.

- Tends to be somewhat expensive.

- Someone needs to be present to prepare the food and it should be consumed completely. The food is essentially raw and moistened food should not be left out for an extended period of time.

**TIP**

**Suggestions for improvement:**
- Providing a high-quality omega-3 supplement will help to balance the fatty acid profile.

- No doubt about it, probiotics and digestive enzymes will further support healthy digestion.

**NOTE:** I'VE GATHERED SOME AMAZING EDUCATIONAL RESOURCES TOGETHER. HOW TO ACCESS THEM IS FOUND IN THE RESOURCES CHAPTER.

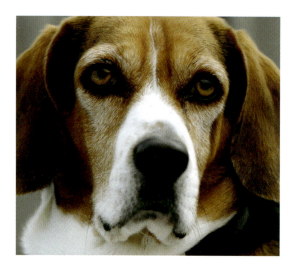

 **#5** **Canned dog foods. Found in health food stores/pet stores/ grocery stores/online**

**Pros:**

- Convenient
- Shelf stable
- Higher moisture content than dry food
- Relatively inexpensive as compared to frozen and refrigerated foods

**Cons:**

- Research is required to determine ingredient quality.
- If can is opened and isn't completely eaten in one feeding, proper refrigeration is required for higher quality foods.

 **TIP**

**Suggestions for improvement:**
Crucial with canned foods:

- Probiotics and digestive enzymes will support healthy digestion and bring the dead canned food to life.
- By adding in a high-quality omega-3 supplement, you will provide essential fatty acids lost in the canning process.

 **#4** **Refrigerated cooked food. Found in pet stores/health food stores/ many human grocery stores**

**Pros:**

- Excellent moisture density since the foods are only gently heated
- Minimal nutrient loss to cooking
- Fresher than processed foods

**Cons:**

- Research into the company is required since the quality of the food used in preparations ranges from awful to excellent.
- Requires refrigeration.
- Someone needs to be present to feed regularly and proper precautions should be taken should the meal not be eaten in a short period of time, just as with human prepared foods.

 **TIP**

**Suggestions for improvement:**
- Add in a high-quality omega-3 supplement to provide essential fatty acids that are lost in the cooking process.
- Especially needed in the case of cooked foods, adding in probiotics and digestive enzymes will support healthy digestion.

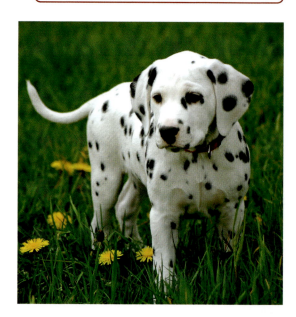

## There are various levels of canned foods available:

**Human-grade – best choice.
Found in stores that focus on food quality like pet boutique stores, health food stores, online**

- When researching food quality, if the company's website doesn't say the ingredients are human-grade, most likely they are not.

- These canned foods will be more expensive than feed-grade or animal-grade canned food, and the quality of the food will reflect that.

- Organ meats, whether or not you are feeding an all raw diet, are an excellent and healthful addition to your dog's diet. It is possible to find a high quality, human-grade formula that includes one or more organ meats in the list of ingredients.

**Premium canned food – good choice.
Found in big-box stores like Petco and PetSmart or a conventional veterinarian's clinic**

- Contain feed-grade ingredients (not approved for human consumption).

- Better moisture content than dry food.

- Many have excellent ratios of protein, fat, fiber and carbohydrates.

**Grocery store brand canned food – worst choice in canned food.**

- Although they contain more moisture than dry foods, they usually have excess grains and toxic preservatives.

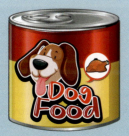

**TIP**

**Important note!**

There are also excellent multivitamin/mineral products on the market these days for your pet. Often all you'll have to do is sprinkle them on the food you've prepared or purchased to be sure that you're meeting your dog's nutritional needs. Some of them also provide living components to support your dog's vitality in the same product, like probiotics, enzymes and superfoods that target the particular needs of a canine. Peace of mind!

**#6  Dry food, commonly called "kibble".
Found in health food stores/ pet stores of all types/ grocery stores/ online.**

**Pros:**

- Shelf stable.

- Convenient – can be offered in a feeder or left in a dish without spoiling.

- Relatively inexpensive compared to frozen or refrigerated foods or even some canned foods, depending on quality.

**Cons:**

- Very low moisture content leading to chronic dehydration and over time a sad variety of health issues as we've discussed.

**Suggestions for improvement:**
critical with dry foods (kibble):

- Probiotics and digestive enzymes will support healthy digestion and bring the dead kibble to life.

**TIP**

- By adding in a high-quality omega-3 supplement, you will provide essential fatty acids lost in the manufacturing process.

- Add water to kibble to increase moisture content.

## Once again, there are various levels of dry foods available:

**Human-grade – best choice.
Found at boutique pet stores,
health food stores, online**

- Best kibble because at least the ingredients have passed quality inspections.

- Very low moisture content (approx.12% as opposed to optimal 70%)

- Unnecessary carbohydrates required to give food its kibble shape

- Best product-baked human grade food – it will be clearly stated on label.

- If no mention of baking, food was extruded (processed with extremely high heat) which means that most likely it contains the residue of carcinogens formed in the manufacturing process.

**Premium dry food– good choice
Found at health food stores, boutique pet stores, conventional veterinary clinics and big-box stores**

- Made with feed-grade ingredients not approved for humans

- Extremely low moisture content

- In most cases, naturally preserved which is a good thing

- Extruded, so the food may contain the residue of carcinogens

- Unnecessary carbohydrates to maintain kibble shape

- May contain or grow molds that can cause health issues for your dog. Be sure and check the expiration date. For safety no food should be kept longer than a year from manufacture date.

**Grocery store brand dry food –
worst choice in dry food**

- Extremely low moisture content

- Contain excess grains

- Contains toxic preservatives

 **Semi-moist pouched food**

**Terrible for your dog** – besides excess carbs and toxic preservatives, can also contain propylene glycol (closely related to anti-freeze) in order to retain moisture – **AVOID!**

 **Unbalanced raw or cooked homemade diet**

It may surprise you to see this category as the worst possible diet for your beloved pet. Didn't we say that fresh, homemade food is a good thing? Yes, we did, if you as a responsible pet parent have taken the time to really understand your dog's nutritional requirements! It's immensely disturbing to learn after speaking with veterinarians that some well-intended pet guardians, feeding their dog a limited diet, day after day, of chicken breast and veggies as their daily meals, have caused irreversible and even fatal health issues for their best friends.

This happens due to nutritional deficiencies and imbalances caused by lack of education on the part of the well-intentioned pet parent. Appropriate recipes for your dog considering breed and age are essential for complete nutritional balance. Issues that can arise include endocrine dysfunction, skeletal problems, and organ degeneration resulting from deficiencies in calcium, various trace minerals and essential fatty acids. I don't want this to happen to you and your beloved dog. Daily homemade diets must be done correctly as we've mentioned.

 **Adding a scoop of a vitamin/ mineral/ superfood supplement to your dog's daily diet is a great idea to be sure that you're both safe, rather than sorry.**

**I offer you excellent education links in our Resources section to help you provide optimum nutrition for your beloved pet.**

Realistically, most of you who are reading this will most likely be feeding your dog food that you purchased in some sort of pet food store, health food store, grocery store or online. You'll be happy to learn that as long as your dog food choice says on the label "AAFCO compliant", it contains at least minimum vitamin and mineral requirements for your dog to survive. That's a start. It's also a very good idea to look for the statement "Made in the USA".

If today you are unable to provide your dog with the quality of food that you would ultimately like to offer for any of the factors we've discussed, perhaps you can make a goal to take small steps toward upgrading your next bag or cans of food, or even offering one or two wholesome, home prepared meals weekly. The great news is, adding in any meals (or wholesome treats) with higher quality ingredients and/or moisture content is an excellent step toward a longer and healthier life for your four-legged companion.

---

**Easily learn about AAFCO and understand nutritional information presented on dog food labels from links provided in the Resources section.**

---

**PLEASE DON'T MIX A RAW MEAL WITH KIBBLE!** THE FOOD TYPES ARE DIGESTED DIFFERENTLY AND MIXING THEM IN ONE MEAL COULD CAUSE DIGESTIVE ISSUES. **OFFER RAW FOODS AND TREATS OR GENTLY COOKED FOODS AT ONE FEEDING TIME, AND KIBBLE AT A DIFFERENT MEAL.**

## The Bottom Line on "Treats"

Commercially manufactured treats may be the worst enemy of your dog's health and vitality!

**Here's the good news** – replacing store-bought manufactured treats with wholesome, moisture rich and nutrient dense, fresh treats to any dog's diet can make a very positive impact on their overall health! Please remember, as with your own diet, regarding treats – moderation is the key!

**Check out this list of easy to purchase, healthy treats for you and your best friend:**

**Fruits:**
- Watermelon
- Blueberries
- Apples
- Cantaloupe
- Bananas

**Veggies:**
- Carrots
- Green beans
- Asparagus
- Sweet potatoes
- Pumpkin

And for even more fun, you can quickly make celery stuffed with plain almond or peanut butter. Please be sure that nut butters do not contain xylitol which can cause life-threatening toxicity for your pet. One half of a stuffed celery treat per day is great for your companion. Perhaps you'd like to enjoy the other half yourself.

As for meats as treats, there are many jerky type treats available to purchase, even at your local grocery store. Look for products that list only one ingredient. For example – dehydrated chicken, dehydrated beef or dehydrated bison. As with food, look for "Made in the USA" on the label.

## Guaranteed Analysis

| | | | |
|---|---|---|---|
| Crude Protein (Min) | 25% | Selenium (Min) | 0.3mg/kg |
| Crude Fat (Min) | 8% | Vitamin A (Min) | 15000 IU/kg |
| Crude Fat (Max) | 12% | Vitamin E (Min) | 460 IU/kg |
| Crude Fiber (Max) | 5.5% | Ascorbic Acid* (Min) | 70mg/kg |
| Moisture (Max) | 12% | Glucosamine* (Min) | 400ppm |
| Linoleic Acid (Min) | 1.3% | | |
| Calcium (Ca) (Min) | 0.9% | | |
| Phosphorus (P) (Min) | 0.7% | | |

*Not recognized as an essential nutrient by the AAFCO Dog Nutrient Profiles

## A Few Tips on Reading Dog Food Labels

As we've discussed in previous chapters in this book, over-consumption of carbohydrates is often responsible for obesity and age-related disorders in your pet. Interestingly, the carbohydrate content is not even listed on most labels of dog food. In a nut shell, this is primarily due to the fact that the dog food industry is self-regulated (a bit like a fox in a hen house) and they have decided not to offer that pertinent information to the buying public.

Even though dogs have no biological requirement for grains (corn, wheat, gluten, barley, rice) dog food manufacturers regularly add in carbs since they are inexpensive and are necessary for the dry food to hold together in a kibble form or a treat. Fortunately, our dogs are very resilient and can process these products, with sad negative health implications only showing up over time.

In wild dogs and wolves, research has shown that the maximum amount of carbohydrates normally processed by their digestive systems is 30% of their diet (from berries, grasses and the contents of their prey's intestinal system). So it makes sense that optimally 30% carbohydrates would be the upper end of your dog's daily carbohydrate intake. The closer to 30% carbs, the better it will be in the long run for your pet. Unfortunately, many kibbles contain 40 – 70% carbohydrate!

In my recent book, Skinny Gut Diet, I offered what I called a Teaspoon Tracker – which helped a person to be able to take a quick look at a box, can or bag label and figure out the amount of teaspoons of hidden carbohydrates (sugars) in a serving of food. If someone had told me that only a few years later, I would be sharing the same type of information for dogs, I wouldn't have believed them!

Similarly to the human Teaspoon Tracker, with just a little basic math we can now figure out the carbohydrate content of dry foods and treats for our dogs. Here's how:

**Look at your label on your package of kibble that says Guaranteed Analysis.**

Begin with 100%.
- Subtract the % of crude protein
- Subtract the % of crude fat
- Subtract the % of moisture
- Disregard the % of crude fiber
- Subtract the % of ash. Often ash won't be mentioned, so use 6% as the common figure.

(**Note:** you will see that maximum and minimum amounts are mentioned. For our general purposes that won't be important)

For example, in the label shown for a Weight Management product (I wanted to look at a product like this since one of the issues with excess carbs is obesity!):

**100% – 25% (protein) – 8% (fat) – 12% (moisture) – 6% (ash – not listed) = 49% carbohydrates**

49% carbs. This doesn't seem like it would be an optimal feeding choice for a dog with weight issues. At least it's better than 70% carbs!

As I'm sure you're beginning to see, By far the highest carbohydrate overload for your dog will be experienced through dry kibble (and treats). There is actually a different formula for calculating carbohydrate content in wet foods that can be explored through a link in our Resources section.

Another important health factor for your dog is the amount of protein and fat provided in a meal. Generally, veterinarians agree that they'd like to see for an adult healthy dog between 18-25% protein along with 10-15% fat content in a food. This amounts to the calories that are provided from protein approximately equaling those provided by fat.

Remember that the requirements can be very different for puppies, older, more sedentary dogs, particular breeds or pregnant moms. It can also get slightly confusing with regarding how to figure this information from a label. Good news, there are some excellent videos available to assist you in determining this important information if you're interested!

**Please visit the Resources section at the back of the book to be directed toward more on these calculation topics to better avoid obesity and age-related issues.**

Please understand this - your dog enjoys sugar like you do! Your dear pet can also become addicted to the taste of processed foods (they too contain sugars) and it may take some time for you to transition them to an enthusiastic response to a more healthful product.

If you are currently feeding kibble to your dog, please be aware that it's very dense with calories, tends to be addictive, and if you leave it out (free-feed), your dog will most likely overeat. If you feed kibble, be sure to limit the portions.

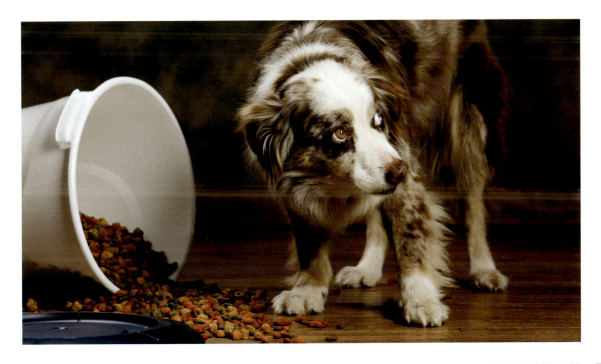

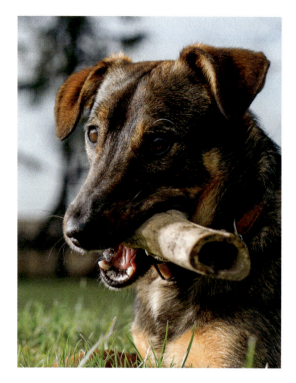

Veterinarians suggest transitioning from one food to another over time, starting with a small amount of new food/old food and shifting gently. Observe which products your dog enjoys and agrees with him or her. There's no hurry, you're both on a more healthful path. Ease of transition can depend on how long your best friend has been "enjoying" his present diet. Perhaps you can remember how at one time you shifted from fast food to a more healthful lifestyle.

**More information on transitioning your dog from their current diet to more healthful choices are available in the Resources chapter.**

What about the actual ingredients on a dog food label? Of course, they will vary by company and food type.

I have some friends who recently started a dog food company. They pride themselves on offering total transparency to their customers regarding the quality of ingredients they include in their products and where they are sourced. To see how they list their quality ingredients, check them out at dogcertified.com.

Here's a short list of info on ingredients to get you started. When you're looking at a label, you want a specific meat (like chicken, beef, turkey) to be in at least the first 2 positions on the label. The ingredients are listed by weight, so you have a better chance at a more quality food when you see specifics meats like chicken and duck as the first two ingredients.

**Do your best to notice and avoid the following ingredients when choosing your dog food:**

- Avoid food that just says "meat" with no particular source specified (an unnamed species). The protein or fat source can be parts and types of animals you'd rather not think about. Additionally, they can be protein fractions from different types of sources (do you remember that you learned that almost everything has a protein component?) Gluten protein is no substitute for real meat for your favorite carnivore – your dog.

- Avoid ingredients like "brewer's rice", "wheat hull run" and "rice hulls" which offer no value for your pet. Dog food manufacturers often use processed fraction remnants like these from the human food industry. Not all fraction remnants are a problem. Should you see "beet pulp" or "tomato pumice" on a more quality food, it's likely they were added as fiber supplements that can be helpful for your pet.

- It's also a good idea to avoid "meal" in most cases – bone meal, meat meal. Meal in general is ground up, dehydrated, and often from an unnamed source.

- Generally, avoid "by-products". Although in higher quality products, by-products can be organs like liver and kidney, when you're evaluating inexpensive products, assume that by-products are low quality.

- Avoid artificial colors, sweeteners and chemical preservatives whenever possible.

**Much more detailed information on the in's and out's of understanding food labels is available through links offered in the Resources section of this book.**

**Busting common false beliefs (I believed some of them myself before I dove into the research for this book!)**

**My dog gets all the water needed for health by drinking out of his bowl daily. - FALSE**

Unless you are feeding your dog fresh whole foods, gently cooked foods, or buying a good quality canned food, the likelihood is that your dog is dealing with mild-dehydration on a daily basis. The great news is that offering moisture rich natural treats (NOT the moist commercial treats) and whole food meals along with lots of clean water can help protect your dog's kidneys and organs against early degenerative issues.

**Dry dog food cleans your dog's teeth. - FALSE**

The carbohydrates necessary to keep kibble in its shape actually add to plaque and decay on your dog's teeth. There are some dry treats that have been specially designed to help clean teeth available at your veterinarian's office.

**Human food is not good for a dog. - FALSE**

Fresh, whole meats, vegetables and fruits are great for your pet, either as a regular dietary choice with certain nutrient additives (already discussed) or as delicious treats. There are many vegetables, fruits and even nut butters that are terrific as treats for both you and your dog. Dogs just like children do not have the ability to pick out a balanced diet from a smorgasbord of food so be careful that the treats are part of an overall balanced feeding plan.

**Treats that mention "meat" on the label contain mostly meat. - FALSE**

In far too many cases, treats for dogs contain little meat and a huge amount of carbohydrates and preservatives.

**Since treats are so small, they can't harm my dog's health. - FALSE**

Even small treats, often filled with carbohydrates, preservatives, corn syrup and other toxic substances can cause health issues over time.

**Grain-free kibble is much better for my dog than regular kibble with wheat, gluten, corn, and/or other grains. - FALSE**

Although grain-free is a better choice than foods with wheat, corn, and other processed starches, grain-free foods are not starch-free. As you now understand, excess processed carbs (and all kibble and commercial treats are highly processed) lay the foundation for inflammation and disease in your dog down the road. Technically all foods sold in the pet store and grocery store that claim to be "grain free" actually contain grain when tested in multiple veterinary studies. This is due to cross-contamination that happens at the factory. Although there are many brands of dog food, there are only a few big packaging manufacturers and the majority of dog foods are processed on the same machinery.

Similar to allergy warnings on food labels for humans that have the disclaimer "The product is manufactured in a facility that processes other products which may contain soy, dairy, wheat, peanuts and may contain traces of all of the above", the only truly grain free foods are either made by the owner or special veterinary prescription diets. This information would be important only if your dog exhibits significant allergic symptoms that you believe are associated with diet.

A well-fed dog, and by that I mean fed and supported with nutritionally balanced and living ingredients, will thank you with increased energy, vitality, and longevity. He or she will require much less veterinary care over time and perhaps most importantly, your best friend will be by your side for many happy years to come.

NOTE: I'VE GATHERED SOME AMAZING EDUCATIONAL RESOURCES TOGETHER. HOW TO ACCESS THEM IS FOUND IN THE RESOURCES CHAPTER.

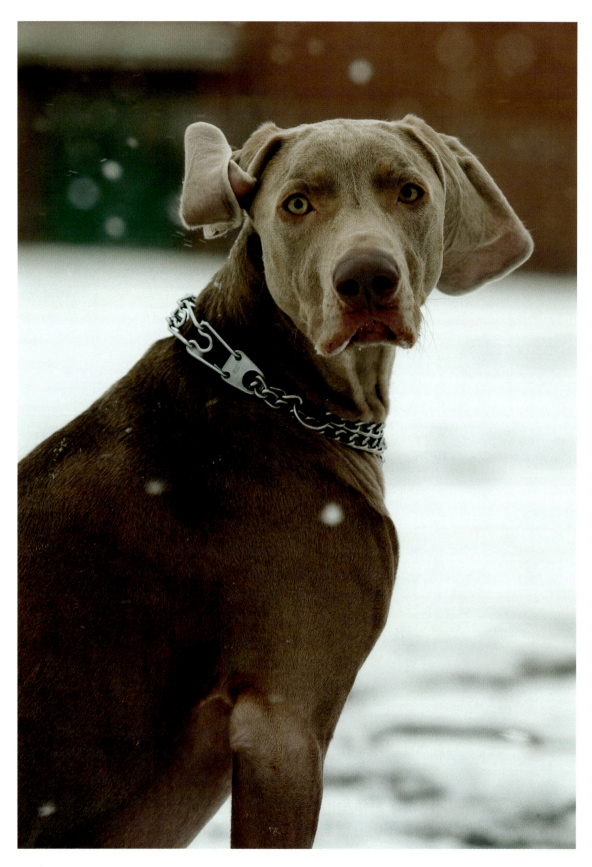

# CHAPTER 6

# DETOXIFICATION –
# FOR YOUR PET'S
# ONGOING HEALTH

Research reveals that the level of toxins in our pets' bodies is significantly greater than that in humans. Dogs and cats experience a higher exposure to pesticides, herbicides and environmental chemicals, mainly because they have more direct contact with toxins than people do. Indoors, they often chew and lay on chemically treated carpets and floors. They absorb a wide variety of contaminants through their paws, and if they later lick their feet, those contaminants are then absorbed into the body.

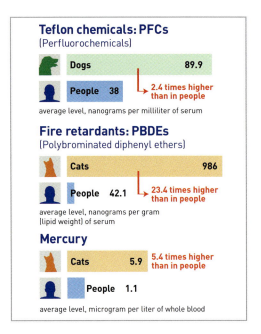

**Teflon chemicals: PFCs**
(Perfluorochemicals)

Dogs — 89.9

People — 38

2.4 times higher than in people

average level, nanograms per milliliter of serum

**Fire retardants: PBDEs**
(Polybrominated diphenyl ethers)

Cats — 986

People — 42.1

23.4 times higher than in people

average level, nanograms per gram (lipid weight) of serum

**Mercury**

Cats — 5.9

5.4 times higher than in people

People — 1.1

average level, microgram per liter of whole blood

In a study conducted by the non-profit organization Environmental Working Group (EWG), scientists discovered notably high levels of industrial chemicals in America's pets. Dogs and cats ingest pollutants in tap water, play on lawns coated with pesticide residue, and inhale both indoor and outdoor air contaminants. Plus, with their shorter life spans, pets also may develop health problems from these exposures sooner than humans might, researchers at EWG said.

Samples of blood and urine were obtained from 20 dogs and 37 cats at a Virginia veterinary clinic, and results showed that the total number of animals were contaminated with 48 of the 70 industrial chemicals for which the group was tested. The average levels of many chemicals were higher in pets than they are typically in humans, with 2.4 times higher levels of PFCs (perfluorochemicals) in dogs, 23 times more PBDEs (polybrominated diphenylethers) in cats and more than 5 times the amount of mercury, compared with average levels in people. Such manmade chemicals, used often in non-stick cookware, carpets, upholstery and other household items for their flame-resistant properties, have already been linked to serious health risks in humans.

Canine samples specifically were contaminated with 35 chemicals, including 11 carcinogens (cancer-causing compounds), 31 chemicals toxic to the reproductive system, and 24 chemicals toxic to the neurological system. Of particular concern are the carcinogens, since dogs have much higher rates than humans of many cancers, including skin cancer (35 times higher), bone cancer (8 times higher), breast tumors (4 times higher), as well as twice the incidence of leukemia, according to the Texas A&M University Veterinary Medical Center.

**Holistic veterinarians categorize toxins into two basic groups:**

- External Toxins: Toxins that enter the body from the environment by food, air, and liquids

- Internal Toxins: Toxins produced by the body's natural metabolic processes

  External toxins are toxins in the environment that cause disease and disrupt the body's natural processes. Examples of these toxins include:

    - heavy metals such as lead, arsenic and mercury

    - manmade industrial chemicals

    - natural toxins such as those produced by mold and bacteria

- Internal toxins are produced by the body (from diet) as the result of natural bodily functions. One example is Intestinal Toxemia, the third step the Process of Declining Health.

The unique behaviors of domestic pets place them at risk for a higher exposure to chemical pollutants in the home and outdoors. As pets groom themselves, they lick accumulated dust that may be contaminated with PBDEs and reproductive toxins called phthalates. Likewise, dogs that eat scraps from the floor also may swallow dirt and dust tracked in from outdoors that has been contaminated with heavy metals, fertilizers and pesticides.

## PROCESS OF DECLINING HEALTH

**Impaired Digestion**

**Imbalance of Gut Flora**

**Intestinal Toxemia**

**Leaky Gut**

**Chronic Disease**

Indoor contaminants—such as flame-retardant chemicals used in bedding and carpets, and chemicals used in paints, varnish, and even soap and shampoo— are even harder to avoid, and it is recommended that owners bathe their pets (with natural cleansers) and vacuum frequently to reduce exposure.

As you now know not all toxins are the result of manmade toxins. Because dogs like to eat anything they find rotting outside, toxins produced by bacteria are a common cause of disease in our dogs. No matter how careful and responsible you are as a pet owner, your dog can consume dead animal remains or spoiled food in seconds.

**Common sources of outdoor toxins include:**

- Washed up sea life and algae toxins from the beach
- Mushrooms and other toxic plants
- Animals and insects that emit toxins, including lizards, toads and red ants

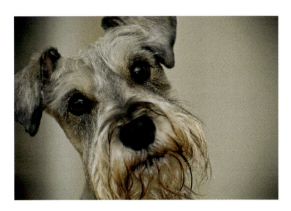

An extremely toxic compound is caused by a species of natural mold called Aspergillus sp. These molds produce toxins known as aflatoxins. These natural, but very dangerous mold toxins represent some of the most toxic compounds known to toxicologists. Small amounts result in acute liver and kidney failure. Exposure to micro-amounts over time results in chronic liver failure, kidney failure and cancer.

## DR. MURPHY

**Signs of Toxicity**

When a dog is exposed to a large amount of any toxin, symptoms are easily observed. There are many toxins, and the signs your pet shows depend on what organ system(s) the toxin affects. For example, any toxin that affects the delicate lining of the stomach and intestinal tract will result in acute vomiting and/or diarrhea. If a dog is exposed to a large amount of a toxin that affects the liver (such as mushrooms) this will also result in vomiting and diarrhea, but also jaundice and often death. Toxins that affect the nervous system often result in acute lethargy, coma or may stimulate the nervous system, resulting in seizures and death. Toxins that affect the kidneys often result in renal failure with signs such as vomiting, diarrhea, mental depression and death.

TIP

Molds grow rapidly in stored dog food. This is why dog food manufactures are always trying to balance preventing mold growth in dog food while at the same time reducing the amount of preservatives in their products. Sadly, preservatives like BHA, BHT or ethoxyquin (among others) have been found to promote cancer and are believed to be generally toxic to pets.

Typically, when a pet is exposed to a highly toxic compound or a large quantity of toxins, the symptoms are acute and veterinary care should be given immediately. But what about chronic exposure to all of the toxins in our environment and in your pet's food? Usually the symptoms are so mild or absent that most pet owners do not recognize the danger and damage to their four-legged friend. These toxins build up in the body slowly, poisoning the cells. Slowly these toxins disrupt the normal healthy function of the cells, resulting in chronic debilitating issues often invisible to the pet guardian.

## THE TOXINS YOU CAN'T OBSERVE OFTEN CAUSE THE MOST DAMAGE!

A dog's body, just like our bodies, is very resilient and can function when exposed to toxins for a long time. Until 90 percent of a dog's liver is destroyed, very few symptoms are observed. Until 75 to 80 percent of the kidneys are destroyed, no obvious symptoms are observed. This is why progressive holistic veterinarians do complete biochemical blood tests on older pets to detect damage before it is too late.

Take for example dental tarter and gingivitis. When a pet has gingivitis, billions of harmful bacteria are injected into the gums, resulting in chronic exposure to bacterial toxins every day. Most dogs show no symptoms while these bacteria and bacterial toxins slowly destroy their kidneys. By the time even blood tests can detect the damage, over 70 percent of the kidneys are destroyed. As we mentioned earlier in the book, that is why your veterinarian is so insistent on routine dental cleaning and care.

In cases of acute toxicity, the harmful effects can be readily observed, such as the recent melamine toxicity in pet foods that resulted in kidney failure, or the occurrence of seizures due to toxic over-the-counter flea products. It's really important for the responsible pet guardian to also consider the harmful effects of slow, and low exposure to toxins on a daily basis.

These cumulative toxins have a tremendous effect on your pet's health. Your pet's body did not evolve in such a toxic environment, and the buildup of toxins in your pet's body effects the function of every cell, often resulting in behaviors that a loving pet parent many times accepts as "my dog is just getting older". Age does not have to mean decreased vitality!

Reducing daily exposure to toxins can greatly improve your pet's health and greatly reduce your veterinary costs.

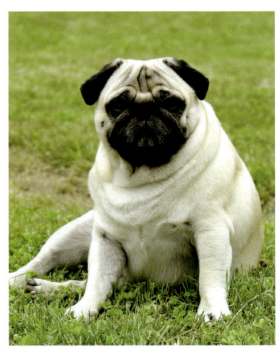

# THE PROCESS OF
# DETOXIFICATION AND ELIMINATION

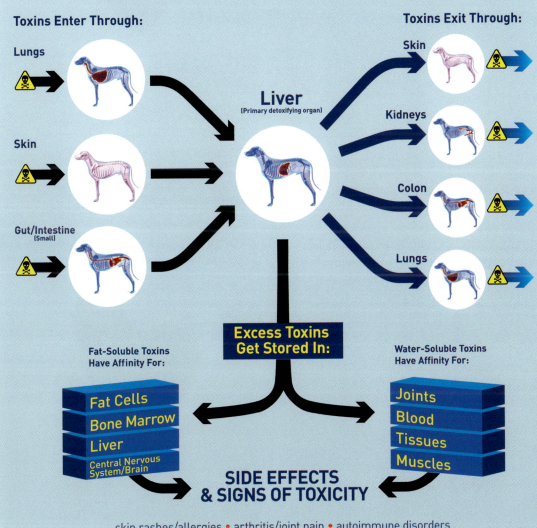

**Toxins Enter Through:**

Lungs

Skin

Gut/Intestine
(Small)

**Liver**
(Primary detoxifying organ)

**Toxins Exit Through:**

Skin

Kidneys

Colon

Lungs

**Excess Toxins Get Stored In:**

Fat-Soluble Toxins
Have Affinity For:

Fat Cells
Bone Marrow
Liver
Central Nervous System/Brain

Water-Soluble Toxins
Have Affinity For:

Joints
Blood
Tissues
Muscles

## SIDE EFFECTS
## & SIGNS OF TOXICITY

skin rashes/allergies • arthritis/joint pain • autoimmune disorders
• constipation • diabetes • diarrhea • inflammatory disorders • IBS
• neurologic disorders • obesity/overweight

Chronic, low-grade exposure to toxins is just as dangerous as acute toxicity, but everything happens in such slow motion that the symptoms are usually never observed and often mistaken for aging problems.

**Such symptoms include:**

- Lethargy and lack of energy
- Dull, dry hair/coat
- Kidney failure
- Liver disease
- Arthritis
- Thyroid disease
- Neurologic degeneration
- Cancer

## Liver Health Is the Foundation for a Healthy Pet

Healthy liver function is essential for overall wellness. The liver utilizes all of the nutrients absorbed from our food to build the vital proteins that are building blocks for healthy body tissue, as you learned in Chapter 1.

**A short review of some of the functions of the liver:**

- Major manufacturing plant for the entire body
- Plays an important role in glucose (blood sugar) and energy metabolism
- Filters and helps eliminate all of the natural and unnatural toxins in the body through a process known as Phase 1 and Phase 2 detoxification
- Metabolizes drugs and toxins and then secretes those metabolites into a fluid called bile, which then enters the intestinal tract so that it can be removed from the body in the stool

## Liver Detoxification Simplified

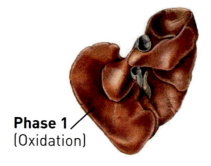

**Phase 1** (Oxidation)

**Liver enzymes process all materials that aren't nutrients.**

**The results of this process are:**
- Harmless materials
- Potentially liver-damaging free radicals produced from oxidation

**The liver protects itself by:**
- Internal anti-oxidants such as glutathione
- Quickly processing materials from Phase 1 into Phase 2

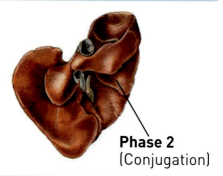

**Phase 2** (Conjugation)

**Liver cells add a substance to the toxin to make it less harmful like:**
- The amino acids glycine or cysteine
- A sulphur molecule

**The toxin becomes water-soluble so it can be excreted out of the body as:**
- Bile from the liver through special bile ducts that carry the toxin into the intestines to be excreted
- Urine, which is excreted by the kidneys

Nowadays the liver is subjected to more harsh contaminants than ever, putting added strain on this already overworked organ.

It's important to note that the traditional medical community doesn't have effective prescription medications that support liver function.

# DR. MURPHY
# ON DETOXIFICATION

The word "detox" is used commonly in holistic medicine, but nowadays it has become so overused that many people are confused about exactly what it means. In traditional allopathic medicine the word was used in reference to specific toxins such as lead (i.e. lead poisoning). Lead can be measured by blood analysis, and then a drug called calcium versonate could be administered, which would then bind with the lead so that it could be excreted in the kidneys. The level of lead could then be measured and a quantifiable reduction in lead could be observed in the patient. When most veterinarians and doctors use the word detox, they are referring to the removal of a specific, measurable toxin from the body.

In holistic medicine, the term "detox" is used in a more general way and does not always quantify the specific toxins involved, prompting conventional doctors to view this definition with suspicion. The more progressive doctors use the word "toxins" to refer to all of the cumulative substances either ingested, inhaled or by-products of body functions that reduce the vitality and health of the body. Because there are so many of these toxins in our pets' bodies, it is not realistic or even financially feasible to focus on testing and measuring each toxin. Instead it is better to focus on gently helping the pet's body in reducing these cumulative toxins as quickly as possible.

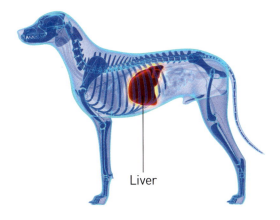

Liver

Fortunately, there are many natural herbal therapies and nutraceuticals that can help the liver efficiently perform its daily workload. When used as a daily supplement, these natural helpers can keep the liver healthy even amid the constant onslaught of toxins in our modern world.

I've been suggesting detox programs for humans for decades. Although many pet owners have been using detox therapies for their own health for some time, they may not have considered the importance of detoxification for their beloved pets.

Since dogs are even more at risk for toxicity then we are, it's critical that their livers are fortified to perform at the highest level in order to process the poisons they encounter effectively. The important question becomes "How can I help my dog detoxify?" Fortunately, detox strategies for dogs are designed in much the same way as I've offered for humans for decades. The goal is to safely assist the liver to do its tremendous job while supporting all the other bodily functions.

Of course, holistic veterinarians have been focused on this area of preventative medicine for a long time.

I've learned that in traditional veterinary medicine, preventative care is primarily focused on preventing internal parasites, external parasites, heartworms, and preventing fatal viral and bacterial infections, as well as nutrition and weight control. Veterinary medicine approaches toxins reactively rather than proactively. When a pet is presented with signs of toxicity, specific diagnostic testing for a single, specific toxin is performed and therapy is then started.

The concept of cumulative body toxins and detoxification is still a new concept to many veterinarians. Most veterinary schools and continuing education programs do not focus on the physiological effects that the massive increase in industrial chemicals and other toxins have on our pets' bodies. The concept of reducing the damage that daily exposure to toxins from the environment, foods, medicine, bacteria, and molds cause is not usually discussed in veterinary schools.

There is no question or debate in both holistic and conventional veterinary medicine that certain herbs and holistic therapies have a protective and beneficial effect on the organs that are responsible for removing toxins from the body. In many research studies, nutritional and herbal therapies have been shown to be very protective against toxins.

For instance, one study involving a group of beagles that ingested a toxic mushroom called amanita revealed that while 4 out of 12 beagles who did not receive treatment died from severe liver necrosis, none of the beagles died from the group that was treated with a commonly used herbal supplement, milk thistle. The active component of milk thistle helps protect liver cells against toxins. Nor did the liver biopsies of the dogs who survived reveal any necrosis.

Some herbal therapies such as seaweed have been shown in research studies to be very effective in removing harmful toxins from the body through the intestinal tract. For example, alginate from seaweed is a natural absorbent

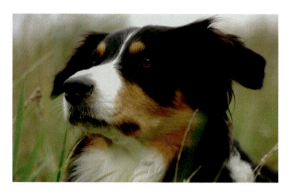

of radioactive elements, heavy metals and free radicals, and it has the unique ability of binding such toxins to its own molecules to assist with their removal. As the alginate cannot be broken down by the bile or saliva and cannot be absorbed by the body, it is secreted from the body together with the heavy metals and radioactive substances.

## A Gentle, Natural Approach to Healthy Detoxification for Your Dog

In the past, you may have chosen an intense detoxification program for your own body where you experienced symptoms of nausea, diarrhea, headaches and general body discomfort as toxins were rapidly eliminated. Although this can be helpful in our fast-paced society where jobs and obligations require you to hurry your own detoxification practices, there is another way to detox for your companion animal which may take a bit longer but avoids most of the uncomfortable symptoms.

As responsible pet guardians, I believe it is in the best interest of your dog to choose a gentle, natural daily detoxification program. As you utilize the power of herbs and other beneficial nutraceuticals, you'll provide safe and effective daily support for each of your dog's organs and organ systems involved with detoxification.

Subtle or vibrational therapy with flower essences are also very important in removing toxins on a sub-atomic level. In many cases vibrational therapies such flower essences work when every other therapy fails. These therapies can also reduce the harmful effects of emotions and stress, which have been shown to inhibit healthy metabolic and detoxification functions.

## Herbal and Nutraceutical Therapies for Gentle Daily Detoxification

### Citrus bioflavonoids
Research shows that bioflavonoids have a great range of medicinal actions including antiviral, anti-inflammatory, antioxidant and antitumor properties. They also help your dog's body to get the best effect from the vitamin C consumed. With regard to the liver, they aid in Phase I detoxification.

### Milk Thistle (silymarin)
Milk thistle has been used medicinally for more than 2,000 years, most commonly for the treatment of liver and gall bladder disorders. A flavonoid complex called silymarin can be extracted from the seeds of milk thistle and is believed to be the biologically active component, one that has a protective effect on the liver. Milk thistle is used to treat conditions such as hepatitis (liver inflammation) and cirrhosis of the liver, and its natural protective properties help safeguard the liver from the harmful effects of toxins and drugs.

### MSM
Found in most plant and animal tissue, MSM is a nutraceutical with anti-inflammatory properties. MSM is a source of natural sulfur which aids in liver detoxification, specifically Phase II.

### Choline
Choline is a constituent of phosphatidylcholine (PC), which is a component of cell walls and membranes. It is involved in fat and cholesterol metabolism and transport, which is important because many toxins are fat soluble and thus stored in your pet's fat cells.

### Turmeric (curcumin)
Turmeric (Curcuma longa) has long been used in traditional Asian medicine to treat gastrointestinal upset, arthritic pain, and low energy or fatigue. Clinical research has demonstrated the anti-inflammatory, antioxidant, and anti-cancer properties of turmeric and its beneficial constituent, curcumin.

Curcumin is responsible for the bright yellow color of turmeric and is believed to be the principal pharmacological agent.

### Flower Essences
Flower essences help to purge all of the emotional toxins that get trapped in the body. While these may seem harmless, research studying the mind-body connection in the last two decades has found that the state of emotional health has a profound effect on the body's immune system and its ability to respond to toxins.

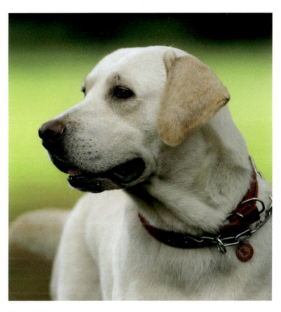

### Lecithin
Lecithin assists the process of fat metabolism in the liver. Lecithin may also improve insulin sensitivity, thereby reducing fatty liver. Researchers believe it may provide a treatment for pre-diabetes, a precursor to liver issues.

### Chlorella
Chlorella is rich in the powerful detoxifier chlorophyll and contains a healthy dose of vitamins, minerals and amino acids, and high levels of protein.

**Ultimately, providing your dog with a gentle daily detoxification supplement will add years to your best friend's life and happy energy to his daily activities.**

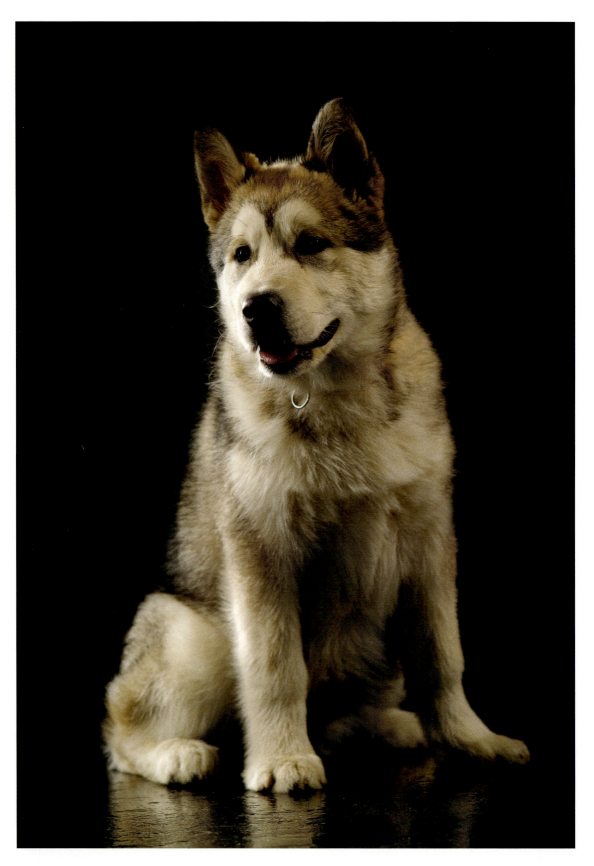

## CHAPTER 7

# RESOURCE AND PROTOCOL DIRECTORY

I'm the kind of person that really likes to hold a book in my hands. Since you're reading this, you probably are too. However, with deeper research, of course the internet is king! While gathering information for this book, and also searching for answers over the last decade for my own dogs, I would like to thank the intelligent people and organizations that have taken the time and focus to create great resources on dog health. No matter my question, there seemed to be an answer, although as in researching human wellness, you can't always believe everything you read on the Web! Of course, your trusted veterinarian will often be your best resource.

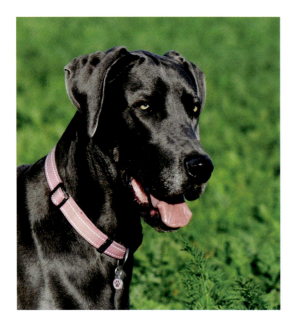

Sifting through volumes of information and choosing what might be most helpful for you was quite a challenge as I wrote this book. I spoke with many people and hope I at least touched on the topics that you find pertinent for your pet. The thought that I could offer this Resources chapter and point you in a direction to delve into issues further yourself was very comforting for me, so here we go.

As in human health care and nutritional needs, there are an incredible number of differing views on what is best, worst and in between. Many traditional veterinarians don't recognize the critical connection between the health of your dog's gut and his or her vitality and longevity.

I find the perfect example of this in the pet world is Pet MD – **www.petmd.com** with a tag line of "vet authored, vet approved". I've found so much information on this site that I feel is extremely valuable, and I've also noticed that there is a huge difference in the views on virtually every subject between one vet and another.

There are so many sites that offer excellent advice, and at the same time may be more conventional in their thinking, from suggestions on how to keep your dog healthy to what food to feed. An example of two of those offering more

traditional information might be WebMD/Dogs - **pets.webmd.com/dogs/** and the **American Kennel Club (AKC) – www.akc.org.**

Sites that I've especially enjoyed that are more focused on natural care for dogs are Whole Dog Journal - **whole-dog-journal.com**, Dogs Naturally Magazine - **dogsnaturallymagazine.com**, and Dr. Karen Becker whose articles can be found at **healthypets.mercola.com.** There are many wonderful bloggers/dog owners that offer their insights on dog behavior and care that I've thoroughly enjoyed as well over the years. And a lot of wonderful YouTube videos created by many pet care experts.

When I offer a resource, please be advised that it aligns with my own natural health care position. Of course, as you will read and research, you will decide in your head and heart what is the best advice for you and your best friend. The information is endless and inspiring. I wish you happy hunting!

**TIP** If I thought that the actual web address was too long to type into your computer, I used an online program called bitly. com to shorten it and make it more convenient for you to access.

## STRESSORS

**Fat Dogs & Dog Obesity: The Facts - AKC**
http://www.akc.org/content/health/articles/fat-dogs-and-dog-obesity/

**How Can You Tell Your Pet is Overweight? - PetMD**
http://bit.ly/2EYBZ92

**Bloat or Stomach Dilatation in Dogs - PetMD**
https://www.petmd.com/dog/conditions/digestive/c_dg_gastric_dilation_volvulus_syndrome

**Anxious when left alone
(separation anxiety) – Cesar Milan** (many
excellent behavioral suggestions)
https://www.cesarsway.com/dog-behavior/
problem-behaviors/anxiety/separation-anxiety

**30 Percent of Dogs Show These Anxiety Triggers
— Are Any True for Your Pet? – Dr. Becker**
https://healthypets.mercola.com/sites/
healthypets/archive/2018/02/12/dog-anxiety.aspx

## PARASITE FACTS

**Intestinal Parasites in Your Dog and What to do
About Them – offered by Dr. Murphy**
http://www.2ndchance.info/parasite-dog.htm

**Parasites and Worms – offered by Dr. Murphy**
http://www.peteducation.com/category.
cfm?c=2+2107

**One of the Least Savory Aspects of Pet
Ownership That You May Not Know About –
Dr. Becker**
https://healthypets.mercola.com/sites/
healthypets/archive/2016/12/17/pet-intestinal-
worms.aspx

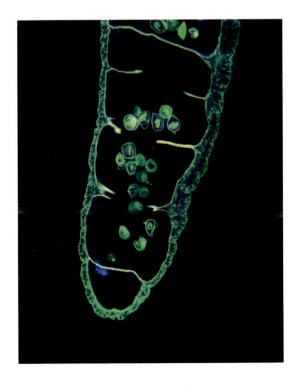

## VACCINATION INFO:

I've noticed that this is an extremely
controversial topic in care of your dog with
an abundance of conflicting opinions offered
on the internet. This is a topic often best
discussed between you and your vet. At the
very least, you want to ask your veterinarian
if they are familiar with titers, rather than
vaccinating year after year.

**Dr. Murphy offers some important
considerations for choosing vaccines:**

All of the vaccines have to be decided on an
individual basis based on dog's exposure and
on what the dog will be likely to come in
contact with. **Just a few of the factors your
veterinarian needs to consider include:**

- local diseases - many virus and bacteria
  are in specific geographic areas
- contact / exposure - pet stores, parks,
  grooming, neighborhood
- home environment - foster care other dogs?
- wildlife around pet - rats, coyotes,
  stray cats, stray dogs
- travel plans
- previous vaccines
- titer results
- likely exposure in future activities –
  boarding, grooming, day care
- previous vaccine reactions
- any autoimmune diseases
- age

**An Inexpensive Tool to Reduce
Pet Vaccinations – Dogs Naturally Magazine**
http://www.dogsnaturallymagazine.com/an-
inexpensive-tool-to-reduce-pet-vaccinations/

**Colostrum and Passive Immunity in Dogs**
http://www.peteducation.com/article.
cfm?c=2+2108&aid=846

## ALLERGIES

**Dogs with Food Allergies: Symptoms, Common Triggers and More – WebMD/dogs**
https://pets.webmd.com/dogs/guide/caring-for-a-dog-that-has-food-allergies#3

**Environmental or Food Allergy? Here's How to Tell – Dr. Becker**
https://healthypets.mercola.com/sites/healthypets/archive/2017/10/21/pet-environmental-food-allergy.aspx

**Pet Allergies to Foods – Part 1: An allergy overview - PetMD**
https://www.petmd.com/blogs/fullyvetted/2007/february/pet-allergies-foods-part-1-allergy-overview-6353

**Food Allergies vs. Seasonal Allergies in Dogs - PetMD**
https://www.petmd.com/dog/general-health/food-allergies-vs-seasonal-allergies-dogs

## DECLINING HEALTH ISSUES

**Small Intestinal Bacterial Overgrowth (SIBO) and Pancreatic Insufficiency - PetMD**
https://www.petmd.com/dog/care/evr_multi_sibo_and_epi?page=show

**Increasing Number of Autoimmune Diseases in Dogs – Dr. Becker**
https://healthypets.mercola.com/sites/healthypets/archive/2016/10/15/autoimmune-disease-dogs.aspx

**Diabetic Dog: Tips to Manage His Diet – WebMD/dogs**
https://pets.webmd.com/dogs/diabetes-dog-diet#1

**What You Need to Know About Pet's Kidney Failure – Dr. Becker**
https://healthypets.mercola.com/sites/healthypets/archive/2016/06/22/dog-kidney-failure.aspx

**Spot the Early Signs of Liver Disease in Dogs - Dogs Naturally**
http://www.dogsnaturallymagazine.com/early-signs-liver-disease-in-dogs/

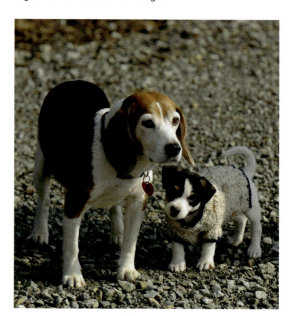

## FOOD CONSIDERATIONS

**Focusing on Protein in the Diet - PetMD**
http://bit.ly/2sL9oiC

**How to Choose the Best Large Breed Puppy Food and Lower Your Dog's Risk of Hip Dysplasia – Dog Food Advisor**
https://www.dogfoodadvisor.com/best-dog-foods/best-large-breed-puppy-food/

**The Best Way to Provide Organ Meats to Your Pet – Dr. Becker**
https://healthypets.mercola.com/sites/healthypets/archive/2012/11/21/organ-meats.aspx

**Raw Bones and Dental Health for Pets / Are Raw Bones Okay for Pets? - PetMD**
http://bit.ly/2onst5Q

**Rawhide Bones and Treats for Dogs: Risks and Benefits – WebMD/dogs**
https://pets.webmd.com/dogs/rawhide-good-or-bad-for-your-dog#1

## CHOOSING DOG FOOD

**Best Dogs Foods – Dog Food Advisor**
https://www.dogfoodadvisor.com/best-dog-foods/

**How to Select a Dog Food in the Pet Supply Store - Whole Dog Journal (video)**
https://www.youtube.com/watch?v=_kVgWoSlUNs

**Choosing Good Foods - Whole Dog Journal**
https://cdn.whole-dog-journal.com/media/pdfs/ChoosingDogFoodPDF.pdf

**AAFCO – official governmental site for the Association of American Feed Control Officials**
http://talkspetfood.aafco.org/readinglabels

**AAFCO Dog Food Nutrient Profiles – simplified by Dog Food Advisor**
https://www.dogfoodadvisor.com/frequently-asked-questions/aafco-nutrient-profiles/

**Carb Counting – How to Calculate the Carbs in Pet Food - Dogs Naturally Magazine TV (video)**
https://www.youtube.com/watch?v=vHONrygcKjI

**Carbohydrates in Pet Food - Good Shepard Pet Food (video)**
https://www.youtube.com/watch?v=1tZSqLt3qkQ

**Topic: Protein-to-fat ratio**
https://www.dogfoodadvisor.com/choosing-dog-food/ideal-dog-food/

**Dr. Becker Shares Her Updated List of Best and Worst Pet Foods (video)**
https://www.youtube.com/watch?v=v0lFwdNm_Go

## RAW FOOD FOR YOUR DOG?

I wanted to offer you some information I found helpful since this seems to be a hot topic these days, and also one that requires a learning curve.

**Why Feed Raw? – Dogs Naturally Magazine**
http://www.dogsnaturallymagazine.com/why-feed-raw/

**Species-Appropriate Diet: Should Your Pet Do This? – Dr. Becker**
https://healthypets.mercola.com/sites/healthypets/archive/2013/04/01/raw-food-diet-part-1.aspx

**8 Benefits of Feeding a Partial Raw Diet - Keep the Tail Wagging**
https://keepthetailwagging.com/8-benefits-of-feeding-a-partial-raw-diet/

**Raw Feeding Made Easy: How to Make A Raw Dog Food – Dogs Naturally Magazine**
http://www.dogsnaturallymagazine.com/early-signs-liver-disease-in-dogs/

**Dr. Billinghurst's BARF Diet – Biologically Appropriate Raw Food**
http://www.barfworld.com/

**Common Raw Feeding Mistakes That Can Be Harmful to Your Pet – Dr. Becker**
https://healthypets.mercola.com/sites/healthypets/archive/2013/04/15/raw-food-diet-part-3.aspx

Clearly, this is only a tiny handful of available resources. Often when you get on one of these sites, you'll be caught for hours reading all the interesting links. Depending on how insatiable your knowledge is for understand your dog's health, the options are endless. Let's continue together to offer our beloved companions their best options for long and happy lives!

**Please be in touch and let me know how it goes for you and your best friend(s)!**

*Brenda Watson*